EVIDENCE BASED WAY TO BECOME HEALTHIER EVERY DAY

A Must Read for Those Who Are Determined to Stay Fit Till 100

Sharad Kumar Betharia

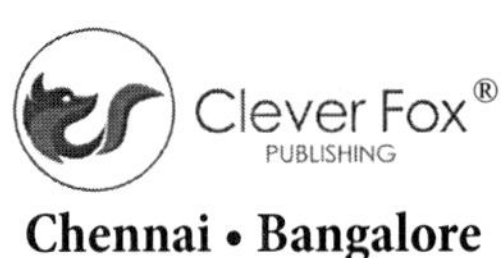

Chennai • Bangalore

CLEVER FOX PUBLISHING
Chennai, India

Published by CLEVER FOX PUBLISHING 2026

Cover Design: By Author

ISBN: 978-93-3443-660-0

"Dedicated to my beloved wife Bhumika, my daughter Vandana, and my son Sandeep—whose unwavering encouragement and support made the completion of this book possible."

CONTENTS

Section 1: Golden Nuggets for a Healthier Life

Section 1

Golden Nuggets for a Healthier Life

Chapter 1
Nutrition and Balanced Diet

"Let food be thy medicine, and medicine be thy food." – Hippocrates

A healthy diet has a profound influence on our body and overall well-being. It impacts every organ system, strengthens the immune response, boosts energy levels, and enhances mental performance. When we eat well, we feel more energetic, positive, and capable of living life with enthusiasm and vigour.

Importance of Nutrition on Health

Good nutrition is the foundation of lifelong health and well-being. What we eat directly influences how our body functions, how we feel, how we age, and how effectively we prevent disease. Nutrition fuels every cell, supports every organ, and shapes our physical and mental performance.

1. Provides Essential Energy

Food supplies the calories needed for all bodily activities - from breathing and digestion to work, exercise, and repair. Balanced meals with healthy carbohydrates, proteins, and fats help maintain steady energy levels throughout the day.

2. Supports Growth, Repair, and Immunity

Proteins build and repair tissues, muscles, and cells. Vitamins and minerals strengthen the immune system and help the body defend against infections. Nutrient-dense foods like fruits, vegetables, legumes, nuts, seeds, dairy, and lean meats supply the raw materials our body needs to heal and stay strong.

3. Prevents Lifestyle Diseases

A nutritious diet rich in whole foods and low in processed ingredients plays a major role in preventing chronic diseases such as obesity, diabetes, high blood pressure, high cholesterol, heart disease, stroke, and certain cancers. Antioxidant-rich foods also reduce inflammation and oxidative stress, slowing aging and disease progression.

4. Maintains Healthy Weight

Proper nutrition helps regulate appetite, metabolism, and body fat. High-fibre foods, lean proteins, and healthy fats keep you fuller for longer and reduce the likelihood of overeating. Balanced nutrition is more effective and sustainable than any short-term diet.

5. Enhances Brain Function and Emotional Well-Being

The brain needs a steady supply of nutrients - especially omega-3 fats, B-vitamins, antioxidants, and quality proteins - to function optimally. Good nutrition supports memory, concentration, sleep quality, and even mood. Poor nutrition, on the other hand, is linked to fatigue, irritability, anxiety, and cognitive decline.

6. Strengthens Bones, Muscles, and Hormones

Calcium, vitamin D, magnesium, and protein are vital for bone strength. Healthy fats support hormone production. A nutrient-rich diet ensures muscle maintenance, better mobility, and reduced risk of osteoporosis and sarcopenia as we age.

7. Promotes Longevity and Healthy Aging

Consistent healthy eating habits improve lifespan and "health span" - the number of years lived without disease or disability. Diets rich in fruits, vegetables, whole grains, nuts, and healthy oils, as seen in Mediterranean and plant-forward diets, are associated with longer and healthier lives. Nutrition is one of the most powerful tools we have for maintaining good health. A balanced, wholesome diet supports immunity, energy, mental clarity, disease prevention, and healthy aging.

Balanced Diet

A balanced diet provides all the essential nutrients carbohydrates, proteins, fats, vitamins, minerals, fibre, and water - in the right proportions to meet the body's needs.

Key Components of a Balanced Diet

Carbohydrates: The body's primary source of energy, fuelling daily activities and brain function.

Proteins: Essential for muscle growth, tissue repair, enzyme and hormone production and immune health.

Fats: Important for brain function, hormone synthesis, energy storage, and absorption of fat-soluble vitamins (A, D, E, K).

Fibre: Supports digestive health, promotes gut-friendly bacteria, helps maintain healthy cholesterol and blood sugar levels.

Vitamins and Minerals: Strengthen immunity, maintain bone and muscle health, and support vital metabolic functions.

Water: A crucial nutrient that aids digestion, nutrient transport, detoxification, and optimal brain function.

Ideal Macronutrient Distribution for a Balanced Diet

Health and nutrition authorities worldwide including the World Health Organization (WHO), the UK's National Health Service (NHS), and the National Institute of Nutrition (India) recommend varied but broadly similar proportions of macronutrients in a healthy diet.

Typically, these fall within the following ranges:

Carbohydrates: 45–60%

Proteins: 15–25%

Fats: 20–30%

For most people in India, a practical and sustainable balance considering food availability, preferences, and long-term adherence is:

Carbohydrates: 40–50%

Proteins: 25%

Fats: 25%

A balanced diet, complemented by regular physical activity, mindful eating, and adequate hydration, is the simplest and most effective path to lasting health and vitality.

The following Food Plate is a visual and practical guide that simplifies the concept of a balanced diet by showing the ideal proportions of different food groups that should make up a single meal.

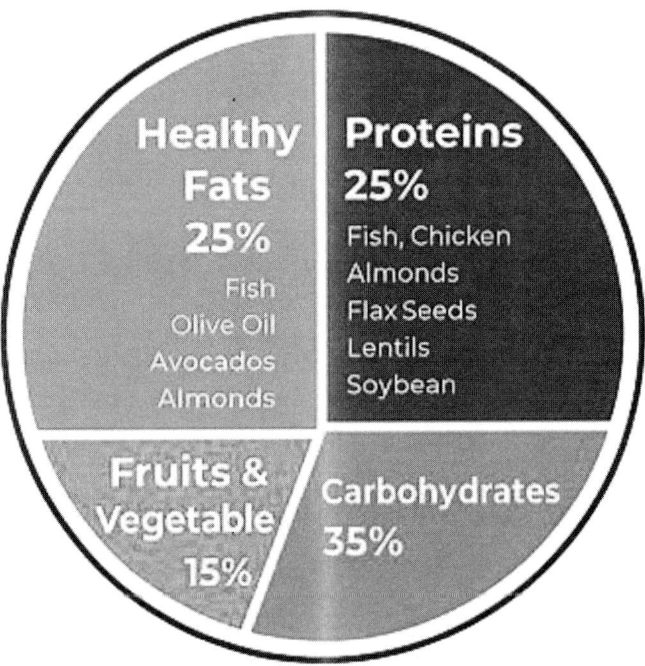

Healthy Fats include Fish, Olive oil, Avocados, Pistachios, Flax seeds, Sunflower oil.

Proteins include Fish, Chicken, prawns, Soybean, Lentils, Almonds, Flax seeds, Chia seeds, Cottage cheese (Paneer), Kidney Beans (Rajma).

Vegetables, Salads and Fruits include Broccoli, Eggplant, Okra, Spinach, Cabbage, Cauliflower, Tomato, Carrots, Cucumber, Peppers, Lettuce, Apples, Oranges, Strawberries, Blueberries, Bananas, Pears, Plums, Pomegranate.

Carbohydrates include Whole wheat bread, Brown rice, Oats,

Quinoa, Corn, Legumes.

Carbohydrate-rich foods are the most plentiful and widely available on Earth. Staples such as rice, wheat, corn, potatoes, fruits, vegetables, pulses, and sugarcane are naturally high in carbs and grow abundantly across diverse climates.

Fats occur in moderate abundance in both plant and animal sources. Nuts, seeds, avocados, coconuts, dairy, eggs, and fatty fish contain healthy fats. Large quantities of fat can also be extracted from oil-rich seeds and nuts - such as mustard, groundnut, sesame, sunflower, soybean etc.

Protein-rich foods are generally less abundant in nature compared to carbs and fats. This natural scarcity is one reason why protein deficiency is common and why modern nutrition emphasizes increasing protein intake. Compared to carbs and fats, protein foods are typically more expensive, less abundant, and require intentional inclusion in the diet.

Food for Thought:

Whenever we talk of plant-based protein rich foods, what comes to our mind are legumes, pulses, oats, kidney beans, chickpeas, etc.

But the fact is that their predominant nutrient content is Carbohydrate and not Protein!

Pulses/Legumes (Cooked):

Most of these foods have 7% to 10% protein (per 100 g cooked weight) and approximately 20% to 25% protein by dry weight.

Seeds and Nuts (Dry Weight):

These plant-based sources are generally measured dry and are highly concentrated in protein:

- Nuts (Almonds, Walnuts, and Pistachios): Contain approximately 15% to 25% protein. Eg: Almonds are around 21%.
- Pumpkin Seeds: Contain up to 30% protein.
- Chia Seeds and Flax Seeds: Contain about 18% to 20% protein.

Animal-Based Foods (Cooked Weight):

Animal products typically have a higher concentration of protein per 100g of cooked weight because they have much lower carbohydrate content than legumes and pulses.

- Fish and Prawns: Lean fish typically contains 20% to 25% protein. Some types of fish can reach 30% protein, but 20-25% is a standard range for lean fish and prawns.
- Chicken, Lamb, and Beef (Cooked): These meats typically have 25% to 30% protein (per 100 g cooked weight).
- Eggs: A cooked whole egg (approx. 50 g) contains about 12.5% protein
- Paneer (Indian Cottage Cheese): Typically contains 18% to 20% protein

The key takeaway is that, nuts, seeds, and animal products are more protein dense.

Chapter 2

Proteins: Body's Building Blocks

Protein is the most vital macronutrient, serving as the fundamental building block for all physiological processes. It is one of the most essential nutrients for human health. It forms the building blocks of every cell in the body and is required for growth, repair, immunity, metabolism, and overall vitality. Unlike carbohydrates and fats, the body cannot store protein, which makes daily intake crucial.

Importance of Protein for Health

- Builds and repairs tissues: Muscles, bones, skin, hair, nails, and organs all rely on protein for continuous repair and renewal.
- Strengthens immunity: Antibodies, which protect the body from infections, are made of protein.
- Supports enzymes and hormones: Many enzymes and several hormones depend on amino acids for their structure and function.
- Maintains muscle mass: Adequate protein prevents muscle loss, especially during aging, weight loss, or physical training.
- Improves metabolism and satiety: Protein boosts metabolic rate and helps keep you full longer, supporting weight management.
- Essential during growth and recovery: Children, adolescents, athletes, and those recovering from illness or surgery need more protein for optimal health.

Protein-Rich Foods

Protein is available in both animal and plant sources.

Animal Sources (high-quality complete proteins)

- Eggs
- Milk, curd, paneer, cheese
- Chicken, turkey
- Fish (salmon, tuna, sardines)
- Meat (lean cuts)

Plant Sources (excellent for vegetarians)

- Pulses and legumes: moong, chana, rajma, masoor, urad
- Soy and tofu
- Nuts: almonds, peanuts, walnuts
- Seeds: flaxseeds, chia, pumpkin, sesame
- Whole grains: oats, quinoa, millets
- Peanut butter, sprouts, hummus

Daily Protein Requirement

As we age, optimal protein intake likely needs to be much higher than the basic RDA (0.8 gm per kg of body mass) to prevent muscle loss. How much protein you need depends on many factors: your age, activity level, muscle mass, health goals and how you distribute it across the day. To support these critical functions, the general recommendation for active individuals is to target an intake of approximately 1 to 1.5 grams of protein per kilogram of body weight. For instance, a person weighing 75 kg should aim to consume over 100 grams of protein daily. Spreading protein intake at every meal, rather than consuming it all at a time is better to maximize muscle protein synthesis.

While this may seem like a difficult target, it becomes entirely manageable by choosing protein rich foods and including protein in every meal and snack. Consistently making smart food selections throughout the day is the key to achieving this nutritional goal.
A variety of sources can help meet your daily requirements, ranging from complete proteins (containing all nine essential amino acids) to plant-based protein rich foods.

Start your morning with delicious Whey Protein Shake

Ingredients:

1 scoop of 80 % Whey protein concentrate.

3 tablespoons of curd (80 gm) or Greek Yogurt, Milk 100 ml, Berries / Banana, Honey and Cinnamon powder.

This drink offers a complete nutritional synergy:

Protein for muscle, Probiotics for gut, Polyphenols for heart and brain and Carbs for energy.

A single shake can fuel recovery, improve gut and immune function, stabilize metabolic health, and contribute to longevity.

Chapter 3

Fats: Healthy, Harmful & Acceptable

Fats are among the most misunderstood nutrients. They are often blamed for weight gain and heart disease, yet some fats are extremely good and essential for good health.

For absolute clarity, fats can be classified into three broad categories:

1. **The Only Healthy Fats – Unsaturated Fats**

Unsaturated fats are the *healthiest* type of fats. They are generally liquid at room temperature and are found mainly in plant-based foods and fish. They exist in two main forms:

- Monounsaturated Fats (MUFA)
- Polyunsaturated Fats (PUFA)

Foods High in MUFA

Nuts such as almonds, pistachios, peanuts, hazelnuts, and pecans contain a high amount of MUFA.
Other excellent sources include olive oil, peanut oil, sunflower oil, sesame oil, canola oil, avocados, and even dark chocolate in moderation.

Foods High in PUFA

Fish and seeds are the richest sources of polyunsaturated fats, especially Omega-3 fatty acids, which support heart and brain health.

Fish found in the U.S. and Europe: Salmon, mackerel, sardine, herring, trout.

Fish common in India: Surmai (King Mackerel), Rohu, Rawas (Indian Salmon), Pomfret.

Seeds with high PUFA are Flax seeds, chia seeds, pumpkin seeds, and hemp seeds.

Other good sources of unsaturated fats are Walnuts and sunflower oil, which contain both PUFA and MUFA.

However, some oils such as corn oil, safflower oil, and soybean oil although high in PUFA, are not considered healthy. These are usually heavily processed, leading to nutrient loss.

They also have a very high Omega-6 to Omega-3 ratio, which promotes chronic inflammation and increases the risk of heart disease and other disorders.

Additionally, corn and soybeans grown in many countries are genetically modified (GM), raising potential health concerns.

Omega-3 Healthy Fats

Omega-3 fatty acids are a group of polyunsaturated fats considered essential nutrients, meaning the human body cannot produce them on its own and must obtain them through diet. They are crucial components of cell membranes and play a significant role in various bodily functions. The three most important types are:

1. EPA and DHA: Primarily found in fatty fish (like salmon, mackerel, and sardines). These are the most biologically active forms.

2. ALA: Found in plant sources like flaxseeds, chia seeds, and walnuts. ALA must be converted by the body into EPA and DHA, a process that is often inefficient.
3. Even if the body converts very little ALA into EPA/DHA, research still shows that ALA itself has independent benefits for both heart and brain health. ALA from flax and chia supports heart and brain health even without conversion to EPA/DHA, because it has its own anti-inflammatory and cardiovascular benefits.

Omega-3s are renowned for their powerful health benefits, particularly for

- Heart Health: They can help lower high triglyceride levels, reduce blood pressure, slow the development of plaque in the arteries, and reduce the likelihood of heart attack and stroke.
- Brain Function: DHA is a major structural component of the brain and retina. It is vital for brain development in infants and maintaining cognitive function throughout life.
- Reducing Inflammation: Omega-3s possess anti-inflammatory properties, which can benefit conditions like rheumatoid arthritis and may contribute to a reduced risk of chronic diseases.

2. Harmful Fats – Trans Fats

Trans fats are artificial fats and the most dangerous type for human health. They are produced by hydrogenating inexpensive oils such as soybean, corn, or palm oil to improve texture, flavour, and shelf life.

Common Sources of Trans Fats:

- Deep-fried foods.
- Frozen and processed foods.
- Baked items like cookies, crackers, cakes, muffins, and pastries.
- Popular snacks such as potato wafers, pizza, burgers, sandwiches, samosas, and vada pav.

Why Trans Fats Are Dangerous?

Trans fats have following harmful effects:

- Increase LDL ("bad") cholesterol
- Decrease HDL ("good") cholesterol
- Raise triglyceride levels
- Promote plaque buildup in arteries, increasing the risk of heart disease and stroke
- Trigger chronic inflammation linked to diabetes, cancer, and autoimmune disorders

You should avoid all foods containing trans fats or those labelled *"Made from partially hydrogenated oils."*

4. **Just Acceptable Fats – Saturated Fats**

Saturated fats are not as harmful as Trans- fats but must be consumed in moderation.

They are found primarily in animal products and certain tropical oils such as coconut oil.

Common Sources are Beef, pork, lamb, chicken (with skin), full-fat milk, yogurt, butter, ghee, and coconut oil.

Health Impact:

A diet high in saturated fats can raise LDL cholesterol levels, which increases the risk of heart attack, stroke, and other cardiovascular diseases.

Therefore, health organizations such as the World Health Organization (WHO) and the American Heart Association (AHA) recommend limiting their intake.

Recommended Limit

Saturated fats should make up less than 10% of total daily calories.

In practical terms, this means restricting consumption to around 12–15 grams per day for most adults.

Summary:

Fat Type	Health Status	Main Sources	Recommendation
Unsaturated Fats (MUFA & PUFA)	Healthy	Nuts, seeds, fish, olive oil, avocados	Include daily
Saturated Fats	Acceptable in moderation	Ghee, butter, coconut oil, meat, dairy	Limit intake
Trans Fats	Harmful	Processed, fried, and baked foods	Avoid completely

Learning:

You can meet your daily requirement of healthy unsaturated fats by including foods like nuts, seeds, avocados, olive oil, and fatty fish in your meals. These sources provide monounsaturated and polyunsaturated fats that help lower bad cholesterol, support cell function, and aid in absorbing vitamins. To incorporate them effectively:

- Use olive or canola oil instead of butter for cooking.
- Snack on almonds, walnuts, or sunflower seeds for a nutrient-rich boost.
- Add avocado slices to salads or sandwiches for creamy texture and healthy fat.
- Eat fatty fish like salmon, mackerel, or sardines twice a week to get omega-3 polyunsaturated fats.
- Keep total fat intake at 20–35% of daily calories, while limiting saturated fats to less than 10%.

Chapter 4

Fiber: Avoid Constipation & help Digestion

Fiber promotes digestion and prevents constipation.
Health authorities recommend a daily intake of 38 grams for men and 25 grams for women.
Dietary fibre is an essential part of plant-based foods that the body cannot digest. Instead of being broken down and absorbed, fibre passes through your digestive system, performing crucial roles that support gut and overall health. It is categorized into two main types based on how they interact with water.

Soluble Fiber

- Action: Dissolves in water and gastrointestinal fluids to form a gel-like substance.
- Function: This gel slows down digestion, which helps to stabilize blood sugar levels and can lower LDL ("bad") cholesterol by binding to it and removing it from the body. It also acts as a prebiotic, feeding the beneficial bacteria in your gut.
- Sources: Oats, barley, nuts, seeds, beans, lentils, peas, and many fruits (like apples, citrus, and bananas).

Insoluble Fiber

- Action: Does not dissolve in water and remains mostly intact as it moves through the digestive tract.

- Function: It acts as "bulk" or roughage, drawing water into the stool. This helps to soften and add mass to the stool, promoting regular bowel movements and preventing constipation. It essentially speeds up the passage of food waste.
- Sources: Whole grains, wheat bran, nuts, seeds, and the skins and peels of many fruits and vegetables.

Most plant foods contain a mix of both soluble and insoluble fibre. Consuming a variety of high-fibre foods is the best way to ensure you get the benefits of both types, which together promote satiety, aid in weight management, and lower the risk of chronic diseases like heart disease and Type 2 diabetes.

Animal based foods generally have very little dietary fibre. So, you must include a variety of plant-based foods in your diet like whole grains, legumes, Fruits, vegetables, nuts and seeds. High-fibre foods include Kidney beans (Rajma), Lentils, Split peas (Tur dal), Black beans (urad dal), Broccoli, Sweet potato, Cluster beans (Gawar beans), Brussel sprouts, Carrots, Chia seeds, Flax seeds etc.

How Fibres Help Digestion and Avoid Constipation

Dietary fibre is an essential component of a healthy digestive system. It is the part of plant foods—such as vegetables, fruits, whole grains, legumes, nuts, and seeds—that the body cannot fully digest. Yet this “indigestible” portion plays a vital role in maintaining smooth and regular bowel movements.

Fibre improves digestion in two key ways:

1. Insoluble Fibre Adds Bulk and Speeds Up Movement

Insoluble fibre, found in whole grains, bran, vegetables, and nuts, absorbs water and increases the bulk of stool. This stimulates intestinal contractions and helps food move quickly through the digestive tract. As a result, it prevents sluggish bowels and reduces the risk of constipation and haemorrhoids.

2. Soluble Fibre Softens Stool and Nourishes Gut Bacteria

Soluble fibre, present in oats, fruits, lentils, beans, and psyllium, dissolves in water to form a gel-like substance. This softens the stool, making it easier to pass without straining. Soluble fibre is also fermented by healthy gut bacteria, producing short-chain fatty acids (SCFAs) that improve gut health, reduce inflammation, and enhance overall digestive function.

3. Fibre Improves Gut Rhythm and Prevents Constipation

By adding bulk, retaining water, and regulating bowel transit time, fibre ensures that stools remain soft, well-formed, and easy to pass. This prevents constipation effectively and naturally—without dependence on laxatives.

4. Fibre Supports a Healthy Gut Microbiome

A fibre-rich diet promotes the growth of beneficial gut microbiota, which play a key role in immunity, metabolism, and digestive comfort.

Adequate dietary fibre—combined with enough water and regular physical activity—is one of the simplest and most powerful ways to maintain healthy digestion and prevent constipation.

Learning:

Soluble Fiber functions as a Prebiotic. It dissolves in water and forms a gel-like substance. It is fermented by the beneficial bacteria in your large intestine. When this fermentation occurs, it selectively stimulates the growth and activity of these "good" microbes.

Chapter 5

Healthy Colourful Fruits and Vegetables

Eating a diet rich in brightly coloured fruits and vegetables is a good way to boost your health. The lovely colour is an indicator of the natural phytochemicals, vitamins, and antioxidants they contain.

Red Fruits like strawberries, cherries, and pomegranates get their vibrant hue from anthocyanins and carotenoids. These natural compounds are good for cardiovascular health, digestive system, and improving eye function. They boost cell function, reduce inflammation throughout the body, and improve circulation.

Orange Fruits such as oranges, peaches, and mangoes are rich in carotenoids. These antioxidants are known for strengthening the immune system, improving heart health, and supporting clear vision.

Yellow Fruits, including bananas, pineapples, and lemons, owe their colour to beta-carotene. Your body uses beta-carotene to produce Vitamin A, a nutrient essential for maintaining healthy skin and sharp vision.

Green Fruits like kiwis, avocados, and green apples contain chlorophyll, a nutrient that is known to help lower cholesterol levels and supports healing processes.

Purple and Blue Fruits: such as blueberries, grapes, and figs, are packed with anthocyanins. These compounds boost memory function, strengthen bones, and support a healthy heart. They are loaded with antioxidants that help fight the effects of aging and disease.

For maximizing nutritional intake, do not discard the skin. Fruit peels contain significant nutrients, so have them for extra health benefits whenever possible.

Red Vegetables offer protection when you eat tomatoes, red capsicums, red onions, red-skinned potatoes, red cabbage, and radishes.

Green Vegetables provide protective health benefits from foods like leeks, beans, peas, broccoli, green capsicums, cucumbers, celery, cabbage, Brussels sprouts, asparagus, and various leafy greens.

Blue and Purple Vegetables give their protection through eggplant, beetroot, potatoes with purple flesh or skin, lettuce varieties with a dark purple tinge, purple or red cabbage, and purple capsicum or cauliflower.

Yellow and Orange Vegetables deliver their protective benefits by including sweetcorn, yellow or orange capsicums, carrots, yams, and pumpkin.

By consuming a wide variety of colourful fruits and vegetables, you can ensure that your body receives several of nutrients needed for optimal health and vitality.

Chapter 6

How to achieve a Balanced Diet?

Achieving the perfect daily ratio of Proteins, Fats, and Carbohydrates (Macronutrients) is quite difficult. Availability of right ingredients as well as measuring of quantities presents difficulties. Having a kitchen scale and a transparent measuring jar are of great help

We need to prioritize consumption of Protein and Unsaturated fats. To get 25% protein, choose protein dense foods like Fish, egg whites, Soya granule/chunks, whey protein concentrate, Almonds, Walnuts, Chia Seeds, Flax seeds, Lentils like Rajma, Moong, paneer etc. You may also add chicken breast, and skinless chicken drumsticks to hit your daily target.

To get 25% healthy fats we can consume Fish, walnuts, Almonds, Chia seeds, Flax seeds, avocados, Olive oil, Sunflower oil, peanut oil, etc. We may also add cow milk and yogurt.

Include plenty of vegetables, salads and fruits like blueberries, straw berries, guava, pears, apple, musk melon, papaya etc. They contain low calories and high amounts of vitamins, minerals and fiber. They should be consumed at least 2 to 3 times daily.

Cereals like rice, wheat, corn, jowar, bajra contain mainly carbohydrates. We don't need to pay special attention to get the calories from carbohydrates. They are an inseparable part of most of the foods that we eat and naturally make up the necessary portion of the diet.

Chapter 7

Estimating calories in daily foods.

We can club foods broadly in different calorie slabs. This helps in quick estimation of calories we consume in a day.

Foods containing 20 calories per 100g:

Tomatoes, cucumbers, carrots, radish, spinach, cooked vegetables (okra, brinjal, beans).

Foods containing 50 calories per 100g:

Fruits: apples, guava, orange, watermelon, strawberries

Milk and clear vegetable soups (Bananas and mangoes are higher in calories).

Foods containing 100 calories per serving:

1 roti/chapati, 2 bread slices, 1 bowl of rice, dal, or sprouts.

Foods containing 200–250 calories per serving:

Chicken/mutton/egg curry/keema/ chicken biryani, Indian sweets like rasgulla, rasmalai, barfi, kulfi, rabdi.

Foods containing 500 calories per 100g:

Fried snacks like namkeen, bhujia, chiwda, and sweets like jalebi, laddus.

Foods containing approximately 1000 calories per 100g:

Oils, butter, ghee, chhole bhature, paneer paratha, butter chicken.

Chapter 8

My typical 1800 Calories Meal plan

It is difficult to achieve the exact ratio of Proteins, Fats and carbs each and every day. However, we should make conscience efforts to choose foods rich in Proteins and Healthy Fats and foods which have good amount of Fibre, vitamins, minerals.

The chart below shows the typical foods for my meal plan for a day. This meal plan has approximately 1800 calories. The proportion of calories from Proteins, Fats and Carbs is 28%, 34% and 38% approximately.

Indian-Style -1800 Calorie Diet Plan

(Approx 28% Protein, 34% Fat, 38% Carbs)

Food Item	**Protein** (g)	**Fat** (g)	**Carbs** (g)	**Calories**
Whey protein (24g)	24.0	1.0	3.0	120
Chia seeds (10g)	1.93	3.13	4.20	54.67
Flax seeds (10g)	1.73	4.40	2.80	56.00
Almonds (20g)	5.28	11.20	4.88	138.40
Pistachios (20g)	5.36	8.80	6.32	124.80
Fish cooked (180g)	38.0	7.0	0.0	210
Apple (1 medium)	0.5	0.3	25.0	95
Banana (1 medium)	1.3	0.4	27.0	105
Oats dosa (1)	4.0	3.0	18.0	120
Idli (2)	6.0	0.4	28.0	132
Moong dal cooked (120g)	9.0	0.4	16.0	104
Cauliflower cooked (120g)	3.0	0.5	6.0	30
Cooking oil (40g)	0.0	40.0	0.0	360
Yogurt (curd 120g)	3.5	4.0	5.0	75
Green salad (250g)	3.0	0.5	10.0	50

Chapter 9

Western-Style, 2000-Calorie Meal Plan

(Approx: 30% Protein, 30% Fat, 40% Carbs)

Meal	Dish	Quantity	Protein(g)	Fats(g)	Carbs(g)	Calories
Breakfast	Scrambled Eggs (2 whole eggs + 2 egg whites, olive oil)	150 g	20	12	2	200
	Whole Grain Toast	2 slices (60 g)	6	2	24	150
	Fresh Berries (strawberries/blueberries)	150 g	1	0	14	60
Mid-Morning	Low-fat Greek Yogurt (unsweetened) + Honey	200 g + 1 tsp	20	4	15	160
	Apple	150 g	0	0	20	80
Lunch	Grilled Chicken Breast (skinless)	150 g	40	5	0	220
	Quinoa (cooked)	1 cup (185 g)	8	4	39	220
	Steamed Broccoli + Carrots	200 g	5	1	12	80
	Olive Oil Drizzle	1 tsp	0	5	0	45
Afternoon Snack	Prawns (boiled)	100 g	24	1	0	110
	Whole Grain	30 g	3	4	20	140

Meal	Dish	Quantity	Protein(g)	Fats(g)	Carbs(g)	Calories
	Crackers					
Dinner	Lamb Loin Chop (lean, grilled)	120 g	28	12	0	230
	Sweet Potato (baked)	150 g	3	0	36	150
	Mixed Green Salad (lettuce, cucumber, tomato) + Olive Oil Vinaigrette	150 g + 2 tsp oil	2	8	5	90
Bedtime	Warm Low-fat Milk	200 ml	7	4	10	90

Total: 2000 kcal

Ratio of micronutrients: 30% protein, 30% fat, 40% carbs

Chapter 10

Top Herbs and Spices for Daily Use

Herbs and spices are among the most concentrated sources of antioxidants and polyphenols on the planet and provide strong antioxidant and anti-inflammatory support to the body. Incorporating herbs and spices regularly is one of the easiest and most impactful ways to boost the nutritional value of your meals without adding significant calories, fat, or sodium.

Turmeric:

Turmeric is rich in the powerful antioxidant curcumin, which has strong anti-inflammatory and cell-protective properties. Regular use helps reduce joint pain, support heart health, improve digestion, and may protect the brain against age-related decline.

Ginger:

Ginger contains key polyphenols such as gingerols and shogaols, known for their anti-inflammatory, digestive, and antioxidant benefits. It helps relieve nausea, improves gut health, reduces muscle soreness, and supports immunity.

Garlic:

Garlic is packed with allicin, one of the most potent natural antioxidants with antimicrobial and heart-protective properties. It helps lower blood pressure, reduces LDL cholesterol, supports immunity, and improves overall cardiovascular health.

Cinnamon:

Cinnamon provides antioxidants like cinnamaldehyde procyanidins, and which help reduce inflammation and improve insulin sensitivity. It is well known for stabilizing blood sugar levels, supporting heart health, and reducing oxidative stress.

Oregano:

Oregano is rich in carvacrol and thymol, powerful polyphenols with antibacterial, antiviral, and antioxidant effects. It supports respiratory health, boosts immunity, and helps protect the body from infections.

Chilli / Peppers:

Chilli peppers are rich in capsaicin, a powerful antioxidant known for boosting metabolism, reducing inflammation, and improving circulation. They also contain vitamin C and carotenoids, which strengthen immunity and protect cells from oxidative stress. Regular consumption may help with weight management, support heart health, and improve digestion.

Thyme:

Thyme contains strong polyphenols such as thymol and carvacrol, both known for their antibacterial, antiviral, and antioxidant properties. It supports respiratory health, helps relieve cough and congestion, improves digestion, and protects the body from infections. Thyme also contributes to reducing inflammation and enhancing overall immunity.

Rosemary:

Rosemary contains strong antioxidants including rosmarinic acid and carnosic acid, which help protect the brain, improve memory, and reduce oxidative damage. It also supports digestion and may benefit heart health.

Fenugreek:

Fenugreek seeds contain trigonelline and diosgenin, known for improving insulin sensitivity and regulating blood sugar. They also support digestion, reduce inflammation, and may help balance hormones, especially in women.

Cardamom:

Cardamom offers polyphenols such as cineole and quercetin, which have anti-inflammatory, digestive, and antioxidant effects. It freshens breath, supports heart health, improves digestion, and may help reduce blood pressure.

Cloves:

Cloves are exceptionally rich in eugenol, one of nature's strongest antioxidants with anti-inflammatory and antimicrobial benefits. They support oral health, aid digestion, reduce oxidative stress, and help protect the liver.

Holy Basil (Tulsi):

Holy Basil contains potent antioxidants like ursolic acid and rosmarinic acid, which help strengthen immunity, reduce stress, support lung and respiratory health, and protect cells from oxidative damage.

Boost your immunity with Golden Pickle

This is an amazing pickle to boost your immunity.

Main Ingredients: 100 g each of ginger-raw turmeric-garlic cloves and green chillis.

Put them in a Chopper jar and chop roughly. Transfer in a bowl. Squeeze 8 or 10 lemons and mix well.

Take 4 tablespoons of mustard oil in a pan. Add one tablespoon each of mustard grains, Fenugreek, Coriander powder, Chilli powder, Turmeric powder. Lightly fry the mix and transfer to the bowl. Mix well.

Now, heat 250 ml of Mustard oil in a kadhai. Let the oil cool down. Then pour it in the pickle jar. Mix well. The pickle is ready. Let it ferment for a couple of days, then store the jar in refrigerator. You can eat one or two teaspoons with lunch or dinner, every day.

The ingredients of the pickle provide:

1. Direct Antimicrobial Support (Garlic and Turmeric).
2. Cellular Protection (Antioxidants from Turmeric, Ginger, and Lemon).
3. Immune Regulation (Anti-inflammatory action from Curcumin and Gingerol).
4. Gut Support (Probiotics).

Regular consumption would certainly provide these nutritional benefits to support a robust immune system.

Chapter 11

Vegetarian Versus Non-Vegetarian Foods

Around 80% of the global population is non-vegetarian. India is a notable exception with over 30 % of its population as vegetarian, due to strong cultural and religious traditions.

Plant-based Foods- Merits and Demerits

Merits: Their cholesterol content is zero. They are rich in dietary fibre which improves digestion and gut health. Good source of vitamin C and phytonutrients (flavonoids, carotenoids, polyphenols, etc.) which protect against chronic diseases. They are generally low in saturated fat.

Demerits: Very low in Vitamin B12 (essential for nerves, red blood cells) and limited in Vitamin D. Some plant proteins are incomplete (missing one or more essential amino acids).

Animal-based Foods- Merits and Demerits

Merits: Rich in high-quality complete protein (all essential amino acids), Contain Vitamin B12 (absent in plants). Good source of Vitamin D (fatty fish, liver, egg yolk, dairy).

Demerits: Lack dietary fibre, have little or no vitamin C and no phytonutrients. Many are high in saturated fat and cholesterol which can lead to heart diseases if consumed excessively.

Chapter 12

Cardio & Strength-Most potent tools for Longevity

Vigorous exercise is one of the most powerful tools for achieving a longer health span and life span. One should be able to exercise at least one hour daily. In fact, seniors who have retired should be able to devote longer time towards physical exercise. A combination of different types of exercises is necessary to provide all the health benefits your body needs.

Its benefits are as follows:

- Strengthens the Heart & Improves Circulation
- Elevates Mental Well-Being
- Boosts Metabolism & Prevents Obesity
- Strengthens Muscles & Bones
- Improves Balance & Coordination
- Enhances Immunity & Longevity
- Builds Confidence & Self-Esteem

In essence, exercise is a form of preventive medicine. It keeps us energized, focused, and resilient across all stages of life.

Cardiovascular Exercise (Cardio): Often called aerobic exercise involves rhythmic movement of large muscle groups over a sustained period, primarily to elevate your heart rate and breathing, thus strengthening your heart and lungs. This type of training, which includes activities like running, swimming, cycling, brisk walking, Trade mill,

Elliptical Trainer etc. is crucial for boosting endurance, burning calories, improving circulation, and significantly reducing the risk of chronic diseases.

Strength Training: Strength training, or resistance training, focuses on challenging your muscles to build lean mass, power, and endurance by working them against a force, such as external weights, resistance bands, Dumbbells, or your own body weight in movements like push-ups, squats, stretches, squats, Lunges, Planks etc. This practice is vital for increasing your metabolic rate, improving bone density, enhancing stability, and making every day physical tasks easier to manage.

Flexibility Exercises: Flexibility exercises are targeted movements, like various forms of stretching, yoga, or Pilates, designed to increase the range of motion in your joints and improve the elasticity of your muscles, making you less stiff and more agile. While it might seem less intense, consistent flexibility work is incredibly important for correcting postural imbalances, preventing common injuries, relieving muscle tension and soreness, and generally keeping your body limber and able to move freely, which is essential for both your intense workouts and your day-to-day reaching and bending.

A good weekly schedule should include 30-40 min Cardio on
5 to 6 days, Strength training workout on 3 to 4 days and Yoga, Stretches or Flexibility exercise daily.

Chapter 13

Zone 2 Cardio-A must for lifelong Fitness

Zone-2 cardio is a moderate- intensity workout performed at 60–70% of your maximum heart rate. It is highly effective for improving endurance and promoting fat burning.

Zone-2 Cardio is simply doing a cardio exercise, like jogging or cycling, at an easy, steady speed where you can still carry on a conversation without struggling for breath. This pace keeps your heart rate moderate (about 60–70% of your max) for a long time, and it's the best way to train your body to burn fat for fuel, make your energy-producing cell parts (mitochondria) stronger, and build a great base level of fitness that makes everything else feel easier.

How to Hit Zone-2?

Maximum Heart Rate: 220 - Your Age

Zone-2 Range: 60 to 70 % of your Max HR

The "Talk Test": You should be able to speak in short sentences or hold a light conversation, but you should not be able to sing or comfortably tell a long story.

Examples of Activities: Brisk walking, light jogging, gentle cycling, easy swimming, or using an elliptical machine at a steady pace.

Zone 2 cardio should be done 3 to 5 times per week. It can be done by brisk walking, running, cycling, stationary biking, Trade mill etc.

Chapter 14

High-Intensity Interval Training

HIIT involves short, intense bursts of exercise followed by brief periods of rest or recovery. HIIT burns more calories in less time, reduces blood sugar, improves heat health. It also increases VO2 Max, which contributes to longer life span.

High-Intensity Interval Training (HIIT) is all about short, hard bursts of effort followed by quick breaks to catch your breath, repeating this cycle several times. For example, you might sprint as fast as you can for 30 seconds, then walk for 60 seconds, and repeat it 8 times. Because you push yourself to an all-out effort, HIIT workouts are short, usually under 30 minutes, and are highly effective for quickly boosting your speed, power, and overall heart fitness.

Most of the Aerobic exercises can fit nicely into a HIIT workout session e.g. Running, either outdoors or on a treadmill, Cycling on a bike or stationary bike, Stair climbing, Rowing on a machine.

HIIT is renowned for burning much higher number of calories in a shorter time due to the intense effort and Muscle Preservation and Building. It also improves Bio Markers like resting heart rate, blood pressure, Insulin Sensitivity and Lipid Profile (cholesterol).

Chapter 15

What is my daily Exercise & Yoga routine?

I devote 90 minutes every morning to brisk walking, strength training, stretches, yoga, and pranayama.

Broadly, I follow the following routine:

Morning Outdoor routine: 6:30 AM

- Brisk Walk (30–40 minutes)
- Pranayama: Kapalbhati, Anulom-Vilom, Bhastrika, Bhramari, Ujjayi
- Stretches for Strengthening Quadriceps (4 times),
- Stretches for strengthening Hamstring (4 times),
- Half squats (30 times)

Routine after returning Home – 7:30 AM Onward:

- Warm-Up (Standing): Standing twists, Hip and knee rotations, Tadasana, Padahastasana.
- Warm-Up (Sitting): Toe and wrist rotations, Cradle, Butterfly stretch, Arm and neck rotations.
- Yoga Asanas: Parvatasana, Ardha Matsyendrasana, Paschimottanasana, Cat-Cow, Bhujangasana, Shalabhasana, Pawanmuktasana, Uttanpadasana.

Evening Routine- 6:00 PM- Strength training

- Dumbbell Exercises (with 3 kg dumbbells- seated on armless chair):

A set of 5 exercises for arms and shoulder which takes 10 to 15 minutes daily.

Chapter 16

Exercises for High Blood Pressure

Exercise is one of the best medicines for high BP. The most recent research recommends following:

Aerobic Exercise

Aerobic exercise (or cardio) should be the cornerstone of your routine. It strengthens the heart and makes blood vessels more flexible, allowing blood to flow more easily and thus lowering blood pressure.
Examples are Brisk Walking, Cycling, Swimming, Skipping/Jump rope. Aim for at least 30 minutes, 5 days a week. Moderate intensity means you can talk, but you are slightly out of breath.

Isometric Exercise

Isometric exercises, where you contract muscles without movement, may be the single most effective type of exercise for lowering blood pressure. Examples are Wall Squat- Pressing your back against a wall with your knees bent at a 90-degree angle. Planks- Holding a push-up position. Handgrip Exercises- Squeezing a small rubber ball or isometric handgrip.

Resistance/Strength Training

Strength training is important for overall health, muscle mass, and metabolism, and it also contributes to lowering blood pressure over time. Examples are Lifting moderate weights, Dumb bells, Resistance band and Bodyweight exercises like squats, lunges, and push-ups.

Yoga and Pranayama

Gentle asanas for mobility and joint movement and Pranayama like Anuloma Vilom, Bhramari are highly beneficial.

Important Precautions and Tips

- Start Slow: Begin with simple brisk walking and increase the duration and intensity gradually. Even three 10-minute walks per day are beneficial.
- Always breathe out during the effort phase (e.g., breathe out as you lift the weight) and breathe in during lowering.
- Warm-up and Cool-down: Never start or stop exercise abruptly. Use a 5-minute gentle warm-up before, and a 5-minute cool-down after your workout to allow your heart rate and blood pressure to adjust gradually.
- Listen to Your Body: Stop exercising immediately and seek help if you experience chest pain, dizziness, or shortness of breath.

Chapter 17

Vitamins, Minerals & Supplements

Vitamins and minerals are *micronutrients* - the body needs them in much smaller amounts than *macronutrients* such as proteins, fats, or carbohydrates.

Despite being required in trace quantities, they are vital for good health, as they act as *catalysts* for almost every essential function in the body.

Vitamins – The Organic Micronutrients

Vitamins are organic compounds that help the body perform critical roles such as:

- Energy production
- Immune defence
- Cell repair and growth
- Maintaining healthy skin, eyes, and nerves

Key Vitamins and Their Functions

Vitamin	Key Roles in the Body	Dietary Sources
Vitamin A	Vital for vision (especially night vision), immune defence, and maintaining healthy skin and mucous membranes.	Carrots, sweet potatoes, spinach, liver.
Vitamin B Complex	A group of eight vitamins that support brain function, help convert food into energy, and are crucial for red blood cell production.	Whole grains, eggs, meat, legumes, dark leafy greens.
Vitamin C	A powerful antioxidant that strengthens immunity, supports collagen synthesis (for skin and joints), and aids in iron absorption.	Citrus fruits, strawberries, peppers, broccoli.
Vitamin D	Essential for calcium absorption to build and maintain bone strength; also regulates mood and supports immune health.	Sunlight exposure, fatty fish, fortified dairy products.
Vitamin E	A potent antioxidant that protects cells from oxidative damage (aging) and supports a strong immune response.	Nuts, seeds, vegetable oils, leafy greens.
Vitamin K	Crucial for blood clotting and bone metabolism; helps deposit calcium properly into bones.	Leafy greens (kale, spinach), broccoli, fermented foods.

Role of Vitamin D & Vitamin B12 during Sleep

Vitamin D stabilises sleep-wake rhythms, supports immune repair, and promotes muscle and bone recovery during sleep.

Vitamin B12 regulates the body clock, indirectly supports melatonin production, aids nerve repair, and ensures smoother, disturbance-free sleep.

Together, adequate Vitamin D and B12 help ensure deeper, more restorative sleep and better overall night-time physiology.

Role of Minerals

Minerals are inorganic elements that the body uses to build strong structures (like bones and teeth) and regulate vital internal processes such as fluid balance, nerve transmission, and enzyme activity.

Key Minerals and Their Functions

Mineral	Key Roles in the Body
Calcium	Builds and maintains strong bones and teeth. Aids in blood clotting, muscle contraction, and nerve transmission. Requires Vitamin D for proper absorption.
Magnesium	Involved in over 300 enzymatic reactions. Regulates muscle and nerve activity, blood pressure, and DNA synthesis. Supports quality sleep and cardiovascular health.
Zinc	Essential for immune function, wound healing, and enzyme activity; maintains taste and smell. Often low in vegetarian diets
Iron	Enables red blood cells to transport oxygen throughout the body, preventing anaemia and fatigue.
Potassium	Maintains fluid balance and blood pressure; supports nerve and muscle function. Found abundantly in bananas, avocados, and coconut water.

Highly Recommended Supplements

While a balanced diet is always the best source of nutrients, certain supplements are often recommended due to modern dietary gaps, limited sun exposure, or specific health goals.

Supplement	Primary Benefit
Vitamin D3	Supports immune function, bone density, and mood regulation. Especially important for those with limited sun exposure, as dietary intake is often insufficient.
Magnesium	Crucial for muscle relaxation, energy production, and heart health. Many people have low magnesium levels; it is also needed for Vitamin D activation.
Omega-3 Fatty Acids	Promotes brain health, reduces inflammation, and supports cardiovascular function. Typically sourced from fish oil or algae; diets often lack adequate omega-3s.
Vitamin K2	Works with Vitamin D3 to support bone and heart health. Directs calcium to bones and prevents its buildup in arteries
Creatine	Enhances muscle strength, power, and exercise performance. Especially useful for those engaged in strength training or high-intensity workouts

Crucial Synergy: Vitamin D3, Magnesium, and Vitamin K2

These three nutrients function as a coordinated team:

1. Vitamin D3 helps absorb calcium from the intestines into the bloodstream.

2. Magnesium activates the enzymes that convert Vitamin D3 into its biologically active form.
3. Vitamin K2 ensures that the absorbed calcium is deposited into bones and teeth — not in soft tissues like arteries or joints.

The Best Way To Take Vit D, Vit B And Vit K

Taking these three vitamins together is the best way for bone and cardiovascular health, but because they behave differently in the body, timing and food choice matter significantly.

The guideline is as follows:

1. Vitamin D & Vitamin K together.

These two work in synergy: **Vitamin D** helps your body absorb calcium, while **Vitamin K2** ensures that calcium goes into your bones rather than your arteries.

- **Take with Food:** Both are **fat-soluble**. They require dietary fat (like avocado, eggs, olive oil, or nuts) to be absorbed. Taking them on an empty stomach can reduce absorption by up to 50%.
- **Preferred Forms: * Vitamin D3** (Cholecalciferol) is generally more effective at raising blood levels than D2.
- **Vitamin K2 (MK-7)** is usually preferred over MK-4 because it stays in your system longer and is effective at lower doses.
- **Timing:** Ideally in the **morning or midday**. Some people find that high doses of Vitamin D taken late at night can interfere with melatonin production and disrupt sleep.

2. Vitamin B Complex

The B vitamins (B12, B6, etc.) are **water-soluble**, meaning they don't require fat to absorb, but they have their own "rules."

- **Timing: Morning is best.** B vitamins are essential for energy metabolism. Taking them in the evening can be overly stimulating and may cause vivid dreams or insomnia for some.
- **With or Without Food.**

3. The Missing Link: Magnesium

If you are taking Vitamin D, your body **must** have magnesium to convert it into its active form. Without enough magnesium, Vitamin D can remain stored and inactive.

- Consider taking a magnesium supplement (like Magnesium Glycinate) in the evening to support your Vitamin D levels and promote relaxation.

Vitamins & Minerals found in Nature

Vitamins and minerals are crucial for health. We should include colourful fruits and vegetables in our diet. They are rich in vitamins, minerals, and phytonutrients that support overall health and reduce the risk of chronic diseases. Strawberries, Blueberries, cherries, grapes, cranberries, watermelon, apples, pomegranates, Tomatoes, radishes, Spinach, cabbage, beets. Oranges, mangoes, peaches, pineapples, musk melon, Carrots, sweet potatoes, pumpkin, red and yellow peppers, kiwi, grapes, lime, avocado. Broccoli, Mushrooms, spinach, cabbage, lettuce, cucumbers, Beet roots, Carrots, blackberries, plums, raisins, figs, Eggplant.

A balanced diet rich in fresh fruits, vegetables, whole grains, seeds, nuts, and lean proteins covers most needs of Vitamins and Minerals However, key supplements such as Vitamin D3, Magnesium, Omega-3, and Vitamin K2 can bridge the gaps caused by lifestyle or dietary limitations.

Chapter 18

My daily Medications & Supplements

Medications Prescribed by my Doctor:

- For Blood Pressure and Cholesterol:

(Telmisartan+Amlodipine) Tablet – Taken daily after breakfast

(Ecosprin + Atorvastatin) Capsule – Taken daily after dinner

- High performance Eye Drops.

Supplements of my own choice:

- Vitamin C 500 mg, chewable – Daily
- Magnesium Glycinate (500 mg capsule) – Daily
- Vitamin (B12+ Zinc) capsule – Once a week
- Vitamin D3 (60k) capsule – Once a week

Chapter 19

Weight Loss - Intermittent Fasting- Autophagy

Managing body weight effectively is one of the most important aspects of maintaining good health and overall well-being. A person having Body Mass Index between 25 and 29 is considered overweight and above 30, obese. Being overweight increases the risk of many health problems, including High blood pressure, High cholesterol, Diabetes and Joint and bone issues.

It's a common belief that going to gym, brisk walk, running or regular workout is enough to shed excess weight. However, science shows that reduction in calorie intake is the primary driver of weight loss. About 80% weight loss comes from eating fewer calories, and only 20% from exercise. When the body receives fewer calories than it needs, it starts burning stored fat leading to weight loss.

The safe and sustainable weight loss target is 0.5 to 1 kg per week. This can be achieved by creating a calorie deficit of approximately 500 calories per day.

Intermittent Fasting (Time Restricted Fasting)

Intermittent fasting is an eating pattern that cycles between fixed periods of eating and fasting. You can fast for 12 to14 hours and eat within a 10 to12hour window. Weight loss & fat burning are the major benefits. It also, lowers blood pressure, cholesterol, and inflammation and prevents diabetes. Eat nutrient-dense foods during eating windows. Stay well-hydrated (water, green tea, black coffee).

Autophagy

Autophagy is body's natural process for cleaning and recycling old and damaged cells, enabling cellular repair and promoting longevity

It is most active during fasting and intense exercise. It helps to slow aging and improve immunity.

Intermittent fasting and High-Intensity Interval Training work together to trigger this process leading to faster cell renewal, improved metabolism, better fat burning and potentially slower aging.

Chapter 20

Importance of Sleep

Sleep is an extremely essential factor for health and longevity. Sleep does some remarkable things for you. It allows your body to rest and perform vital maintenance on your memory, hormones and immune system. Inadequate sleep can lead to memory impairment, increased inflammation, higher risk of chronic diseases, cognitive decline and neurodegenerative diseases.

Sleep deprivation alters multiple systems linked to lifestyle diseases.
-Increases cortisol, elevating BP and blood glucose.
-Reduces insulin sensitivity by 20–30%.
-Elevates inflammatory markers (CRP).
The amount of sleep required varies from person to person. In general, adults should aim to get 7-8 hours of sleep per night. When you are getting adequate amount of sleep, you feel rested and fresh when you wake up.
For getting better sleep, you should follow consistent bed and wake up times, maintain a dark, cool, quiet bedroom.

Vitamins & Minerals for Good Sleep

Several micronutrients are vital for regulating the nervous system and supporting sleep hormone production:

Magnesium: It helps calm the nervous system, relax muscles, and is a co-factor in the conversion of tryptophan to melatonin. It is found in leafy greens (spinach), nuts, seeds, avocados, and black beans.
Vitamin B6, B12, and Folate: These B-vitamins are essential for the body to convert tryptophan into serotonin and melatonin. It is found in whole grains, lean meats, and certain vegetables.
Vitamin D: Low levels are linked to shorter sleep duration and poorer sleep quality. It is found in fatty fish, fortified dairy, and sun exposure.

You should have your dinner at least two hours before going to bed. The major part of digestive process will be over in this time gap, allowing your body to enter a state of true rest when you lie down. In dinner you should avoid fried and spicy foods. You should strictly avoid alcohol, coffee sugary drinks and screens before.

Learning:

Nuts support both sleep quality and muscle rebuilding during the night. A small handful of nuts (like walnuts, almonds, or pistachios) consumed an hour or two before bed works as a dual-action snack: the Melatonin and Magnesium help quiet the mind and induce sleep, while the Protein and Healthy Fats provide the building blocks and sustained energy for muscle repair throughout the night.

Chapter 21

Progressive Muscle Relaxation & Yoga Nidra

Progressive Muscle Relaxation (PMR)

It is a technique involving the tensing and relaxing of different muscle groups for stress relief, also known as Jacobson's Relaxation Technique.

Steps to Practice PMR:

1. Sit or lie down comfortably.
2. Sequentially tense and relax muscles from toes to facial muscles.

Benefits:

· Lowers heart rate and blood pressure.

· Aids sleep and eases tension headaches.

· Improves mental clarity.

Yoga Nidra – The Art of Conscious Relaxation

Yog Nidra is based on autosuggestion**.** It induces deep conscious relaxation at the physical, mental, and emotional levels. It relieves stress, body aches and induces a meditative state. Unlike regular sleep, in Yog Nidra you maintain full inner awareness.

Asana for Yoga Nidra: Performed in "Shavasana" (corpse pose), lying flat on the back.

How Yoga Nidra is performed:

· Lie comfortably on your back.

· Systematically relax each body part from toes to head.

· Shift awareness to visualize your body lying relaxed.

· Imagine merging with the vast blue sky.

· Slowly return to body consciousness, feeling rejuvenated.

Benefits of Yoga Nidra:

· Activates the parasympathetic nervous system.

· Reduces stress and improves stress management.

· Decreases the need for regular sleep.

· Helps in managing high blood pressure, insomnia, asthma, and allergies.

· Brings clarity to the mind and relief from body aches.

. Induces a meditative state

Chapter 22

Circadian Rhythm

Circadian rhythm is your internal biological clock that regulates the sleep-wake cycle over a 24-hour period.
It is influenced by light exposure, temperature, and hormonal changes, especially melatonin and cortisol.

A well-aligned circadian rhythm helps you fall asleep easily and wake up feeling refreshed. You can support Circadian Rhythm by waking up and sleeping at fixed times, limiting caffeine and alcohol especially in the evening and creating a sleep-friendly cool, dark and quiet environment. Disruptions can lead to insomnia, daytime fatigue, and poor concentration.

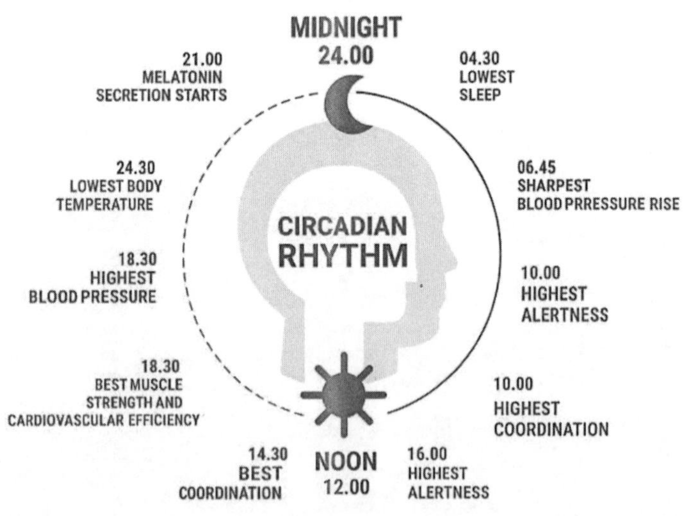

It should be understood that circadian rhythm is definitely different for different people. While the underlying mechanism is the same - a cycle of about 24 hours regulated by light, the timing and preference for sleep and activity vary significantly from person to person.

Some people are Larks (Morning People). They wake up early 5 to 7 AM, feel most energetic and productive in the morning, and go to bed early 9 to 10 PM. Their core body temperature and cortisol levels peak earlier in the day.

Some people are Owls (Evening People). They wake up late 9 to11AM, have their peak alertness and productivity in the late afternoon and evening, and go to bed late 1to 2 AM. Their core body temperature and cortisol levels peak later in the day.

Aligning the day's tasks with your natural circadian rhythm improves Optimal Sleep Quality Metabolic Health, Glucose Regulation, Stronger Immunity, Peak Mental Performance, Improved Focus and Productivity

Chapter 23

Mindfulness: A Guide to Stress-Free Living

Mindfulness is the practice of purposely focusing your attention on the present moment and acknowledging your thoughts, feelings, bodily sensations, and surrounding environment without interpretation or judgment. It’s about observing the present moment rather than being caught up in regrets about the past or worries about the future.

Practising Mindfulness in Everyday Activities:

Mindful Eating

-Eating slowly without TV or phone.

-Savouring the taste, texture, aroma, and chewing consciously instead of rushing.

Mindful Walking

Feeling each step, the ground beneath your feet, rhythm of movement, wind on skin, sounds around you — instead of walking lost in thought.

Mindful Listening

-Listening to someone with full attention, without interrupting, planning a reply, or judging.

-Hearing the tone, emotions, and meaning with presence.

Mindful Showering

-Feeling the warmth of water, scent of soap, sound of droplets.

-Being fully present rather than planning the day in your head.

Mindful Breathing

-Taking a few slow breaths and noticing the air entering and leaving the body.

-Just observing the sensation of breathing without trying to change it.

How Mindfulness Benefits Our Life?

Practicing mindfulness can bring noticeable positive changes. Scientific research strongly supports its role in emotional well-being, cognitive performance, and physical health.

Reduces Stress and Anxiety

Mindfulness lowers cortisol levels and helps the mind slow down. It allows us to observe stressful thoughts without getting entangled in them, reducing anxiety and promoting peace.

Improves Focus and Mental Clarity

When the mind stops wandering, concentration improves. Mindfulness strengthens attention span, enhances memory, and improves decision-making.

Emotional Balance and Better Relationships

With mindful awareness, we respond instead of reacting. This leads to calm communication, empathy, reduced irritability, and healthier relationships at home and work.

Greater Happiness and Life Satisfaction

A mindful person experiences life more vividly—tasting food fully, listening deeply and walking with awareness. Ordinary moments become rich and meaningful, increasing gratitude and joy.

Enhanced Physical Health

Studies show that regular mindfulness practice can: lower blood pressure, reduce chronic pain, improve sleep quality and boost immunity.

What is Body scan Meditation?

Body Scan Meditation is a mindfulness practice where you gently move your attention through different parts of your body, noticing sensations without judgment. It helps release tension, improve awareness, and foster relaxation.

How to Practice Body Scan Meditation (Step-by-Step)?

1. Find a quiet space – Sit or lie down comfortably.
2. Close your eyes – Take a few deep breaths to settle.
3. Start at the top – Begin with your head, noticing sensations (warmth, tightness, tingling).
4. Move slowly downward – Shift attention to shoulders, arms, chest, abdomen, legs, and feet.
5. Observe without judgment – If you feel discomfort, simply acknowledge it without trying to change it.
6. Return to the breath – If your mind wanders, gently bring focus back to the body part or breath.

7. End with full awareness – After scanning the whole body, rest in the feeling of relaxation and presence.

Mindfulness is a way of living. With regular practice, it helps us slow down, think clearly, feel deeply, and live consciously. It reduces stress, improves emotional and physical well-being, sharpens focus, and creates inner peace that radiates into every aspect of life.

Chapter 24

My Bedtime Ritual

My routine starts 30 to 60 Minutes before Bed time.

-This sequence of relaxing activities signals to the body and mind that it is time to wind down, promoting the natural release of sleep hormones like melatonin.

- I turn off all screens like Computer, TV, iPhone. The blue light from these devices can suppress melatonin production, making it harder to fall asleep.
- I have a handful of pistachios and walnuts in a small bowl with milk
- I take a quick shower with warm water
- I draw the curtains to make the room dark to the extent possible
- Switch on air-conditioner for a while to cool down the room and body
- I listen to an audiobook or listen to old favourite songs.
- I jot down the jobs to be done for the next day.

A few Minutes before Bed:

Forgiveness Prayer: To let go of the day's burdens.

Gratitude Prayer: To acknowledge life's blessings.

Serenity Prayer: To fosters acceptance and calm.

After getting into Bed:

Listen to soothing old Bollywood melodies by Kishore Kumar or Lata Mangeshkar on your phone. This helps me to drift into sleep within 15 minutes.

Chapter 25

Six Enemies of Health & Longevity

To achieve a long-life span and health span you must manage or eliminate six formidable adversaries. They are known as the "Six S": Sugar, Saturated Fats, Salt, Stress, Smoking, and Spirits (excessive alcohol).

Sugar:

Excess sugar is a major driver of lifestyle diseases.

Men should limit sugar to less than 30 grams per day and Women to less than 20 grams.

Be aware of hidden sugars in sugary drinks, sauces, carbonated drinks, and processed snacks. Avoid processed foods rich in High Fructose Corn Syrup. Limit high-sugar fruits such as bananas, mangoes, and grapes.

Saturated Fats:

These are found in red meat, full-fat dairy products, and many processed foods. Saturated fats raise "bad" cholesterol (LDL) levels in the blood which contributes to plaque build-up in the arteries increasing the risk of heart attacks and strokes. Choosing lean meats, low-fat dairy, and incorporating healthy unsaturated fats from fish, avocados, almonds, pistachios, and olive oil can help keep this enemy at bay. Recommended daily limit of saturated fat is less than 15 grams per day.

Salt:

Excess salt can raise Blood Pressure and overburden the kidneys

Salt is present in processed foods like bread, sauces, and ready-made meals.

Recommended limit of consumption is less than 2.5 grams per day.

Tips to Reduce Salt Intake:

Eat fresh, unprocessed foods. Use herbs, spices and flavour enhancers instead of salt. Flavour enhancers like herbs, spices, garlic, onion, lemon juice, black pepper and vinegar can help reduce the need for salt in your cooking.

Stress:

Chronic stress, a common feature of modern life, has far-reaching adverse effects on our health. It can trigger the release of hormones that contribute to high blood pressure, weaken the immune system, promote inflammation, and increase the risk of anxiety and depression.

Effective stress management techniques such as physical exercise, mindfulness, yoga, bonding with family and friends and spending time in nature can mitigate harmful impact of stress.

Smoking:

Smoking is the most damaging habit. It harms nearly every organ in the body, drastically increasing the risk of lung cancer, heart disease, stroke, emphysema, and many other serious illnesses. Harmful chemicals in cigarette smoke damage blood vessels, reduce oxygen supply, and promote inflammation

Quitting smoking is the single most impactful step an individual can take to improve their long-term health.

Spirits (Excessive Alcohol):

Excessive alcohol consumption significantly harms the liver, heart, and brain, contributing to conditions like liver cirrhosis, high blood pressure, and mental health disorders. Moderating or eliminating alcohol intake and opting for healthier beverages like herbal tea, lemon water, or fresh juices is a much wiser choice.

Chapter 26

Foods for Lowering Cholesterol, Blood Pressure and Blood Sugar

Food	Key Nutrients	Health Benefits	Indian style preparation
1. Oats	Soluble fibre (beta-glucan)	Reduces LDL cholesterol, slows glucose absorption, aids BP control	Oats porridge, oats chilla, oats upma
2. Leafy Greens (Spinach, Methi, Sarson, Kale)	Nitrates, potassium, magnesium	Relaxes blood vessels, lowers BP; improves insulin sensitivity	Add to dal, soups, smoothies, or as sabzi
3. Berries (Blueberries, Strawberries, Indian Jamun)	Antioxidants, anthocyanins, fibre	Improves arterial health, lowers glucose spikes, boosts HDL	Add to oats, curd, or eat fresh
4. Beans and Lentils (Dal, Rajma, Chana, Moong)	Plant protein, soluble fibre, magnesium	Stabilizes blood sugar, lowers LDL, supports weight loss	Include in daily lunch/dinner as dal or sprouts
5. Nuts (Almonds, Walnuts,	Healthy fats, magnesium, arginine	Improves HDL, reduces LDL & triglycerides,	20–30 g as snacks or with breakfast

Food	Key Nutrients	Health Benefits	Indian style preparation
Pistachios)		stabilizes BP	
6. Seeds (Flax, Chia, Pumpkin, Sunflower)	Omega-3s, fibre, lignans	Reduces inflammation, lowers LDL, improves insulin function	Add 1 tbsp to curd, oats, or smoothies
7. Fatty Fish (Salmon, Sardines, Mackerel, Rohu)	Omega-3 fatty acids	Reduces triglycerides, lowers BP, prevents plaque build-up	Grilled, baked, or tandoori fish 2–3×/week
8. Garlic	Allicin	Mildly lowers BP, improves cholesterol profile, enhances circulation	Add raw or lightly cooked to daily meals
9. Fruits rich in soluble fibre (Apple, Guava, Citrus)	Pectin, vitamin C, antioxidants	Lowers LDL, reduces BP, moderates glucose rise	Whole fruit (not juice) 2–3 servings/day
10. Whole Grains (Barley, Brown Rice, Millets, Quinoa)	Fibre, magnesium, B-vitamins	Improves lipid profile, reduces insulin resistance, lowers BP	Replace white rice/maida with these

Food	Key Nutrients	Health Benefits	Indian style preparation
11. Avocado (or Indian substitute: tender coconut, nuts)	MUFA, potassium, fibre	Improves HDL, reduces LDL and BP	Add ½ avocado or handful of nuts daily
12. Green Tea	Catechins, antioxidants	Improves endothelial function, reduces LDL oxidation, stabilizes sugar	1–2 cups/day without sugar
13. Tomatoes (and Tomato Juice)	Lycopene, potassium	Reduces BP and LDL oxidation	Fresh tomato salad, soups, or juice
14. Low-fat Curd / Yogurt	Calcium, probiotics, protein	Supports gut health, modestly reduces BP and weight	1 bowl daily, plain unsweetened
15. Dark Chocolate (70%+)	Flavonoids	Improves vascular elasticity, reduces BP (small effect)	10–15 g occasionally (no added sugar)

Common Nutritional Themes

Goal	Dietary Focus	What to Limit / Avoid
BP Control	Potassium, magnesium, nitrates, low sodium	Salt, pickles, papads, processed snacks
Diabetes Control	High fibre, low GI carbs, lean proteins	White rice, maida, sweets, sugary drinks
Cholesterol Reduction	Soluble fibre, omega-3 fats, unsaturated oils	Saturated fats (butter, ghee, coconut oil), trans fats, fried foods

Chapter 27

Understanding Human Body & Common Diseases

Basic knowledge of your body and the conditions that commonly affect it offers several key advantages for maintaining your health proactively By monitoring key health parameters and recognising early warning signs, you can take preventive action or seek help before conditions become severe. Early Detection is the key to Prevention.

Informed Lifestyle Choices: Having this fundamental knowledge allows you to make much smarter decisions regarding nutrition, physical activity, and avoiding harmful habits.

Improved Communication with doctors: You will be able to engage in more meaningful conversations with doctors and better understand diagnoses, evaluate treatments, and adhere to medical advice.

Confident Management of Conditions: Awareness helps you manage any existing chronic health issues more effectively, which naturally helps reduce anxiety and enhance your overall quality of life.

Chapter 28

Proactive Health Monitoring: Key to Longevity

A proactive approach to health monitoring empowers you to detect potential issues early and take preventive action before they escalate. And early detection is the key to prevention.

By regularly tracking key biomarkers, you gain valuable insights into your current health status and can consult your doctor to make informed timely decisions. This strategy is vital not only for disease prevention but also for achieving good health and longevity.

Key Biomarkers to Track regularly.

Category	Key Biomarkers	Health Significance
Blood Sugar Control	Glucose, HbA1c, Insulin	Indicators of blood sugar control and the risk of diabetes.
Cardiovascular Health	Triglycerides, HDL, LDL	Reflects your lipid balance and the overall risk of heart disease.
Inflammation/Immunity	High-sensitivity C-reactive Protein (hs-CRP), Homocysteine, White Blood Cell Count	Markers of chronic inflammation and the strength of your immune response.
Stress and Metabolism	Cortisol, Thyroid Panel (TSH, T3, T4)	Assesses stress levels and essential thyroid (metabolic) function.
Essential Vitamins	Vitamin D, Vitamin B12	Crucial for immunity, bone strength, mood, nerve function, and energy.
Essential Minerals	Magnesium, Iron	Essential for energy production, muscle function, and oxygen transport.

Chapter 29

Wearable smart devices-Transforming Health Monitoring

Wearable smart health-monitoring devices are compact gadgets like smartwatches, bands, rings or patches that you wear on your wrist, finger, skin, etc. Many of today's wearables are equipped with sensors (heart rate, SpO_2 / oxygen level, ECG, motion, sleep, even glucose or metabolic markers) and connected apps that track, record and analyse your health and lifestyle data in real time.

Wearables are no longer just "fitness gadgets," but have become powerful tools for preventive health, disease-management, recovery, lifestyle optimization, and even early detection of potential issues.

What Can Modern Wearables Do?

- Real-time tracking of vital signs. Most smartwatches or trackers can continuously or on-demand measure heart rate, heart-rate variability (HRV), blood oxygen saturation (SpO_2), sleep patterns, activity levels, and more. This helps you spot irregularities (e.g. unusually high / low heart rate) early, track recovery, and gauge stress or rest-needs.
- Sleep and recovery monitoring. Through built-in sensors, wearables record sleep duration, quality, and changes—info that can help you optimize sleep, rest, and recovery.
- Lifestyle & fitness data for informed decisions. Combined with activity tracking and metabolic metrics, wearables help you monitor

exercise, calories burned, activity levels, steps taken, and overall daily movement — useful for fitness, weight management, and cardiovascular health

- Early warning & preventive health applications. Some advanced wearables now include ECG features, continuous monitoring of vital signs or oxygen levels — helping detect potential heart irregularities, respiratory issues, or other concerns.
- Regular tracking of sleep, activity, stress, HRV, rest and recovery patterns — over months — provides a holistic picture of health trends, helping you fine-tune lifestyle, diet, exercise, sleep and stress management to suit your body's rhythms. This is especially useful for longevity, preventive health and overall well-being.

Examples of Popular Wearable Devices

The current generation of health wearables is defined by enhanced accuracy and a shift toward medical-grade capabilities:

- Continuous Glucose Monitors (CGMs): Devices like the Abbott Freestyle Libre 3 are moving toward widespread use, providing real-time glucose readings without the need for traditional finger-prick tests.
- Clinical-Grade Patches: Adhesive smart patches (e.g., Bio IntelliSense Bio Sticker) offer clinical-grade, continuous monitoring of multiple vital signs like heart rate, respiratory patterns, and skin temperature, often for days or weeks at a time.
- Smart Rings (e.g., Oura Ring): These devices excel in comfortable, long-term monitoring, particularly for sleep quality, heart rate

variability (HRV), and body temperature, providing a "readiness" score for the day.

- Wearable ECG/Blood Pressure Monitors: Dedicated devices like the Withing's BPM Core or FDA-cleared smartwatch models provide clinically validated readings for managing cardiovascular health at home
- WHOOP 5.0 Health and Fitness Tracker — Popular among athletes or health-conscious users, focusing on recovery metrics, sleep tracking and HRV (heart-rate variability).
- Samsung Galaxy Fit3 — A versatile fitness tracker balancing activity tracking, heart-rate monitoring, sleep tracking and convenience — suitable for regular activity monitoring and lifestyle tracking.

Why They Matter?

They show how daily habits, exercise, sleep, stress, and diet actually affect your body in real time. This data-driven feedback allows you to:

- Fine-tune your protein, cardio, sleep, stress, and recovery routines
- Monitor sleep quality, recovery, resting heart rate, variability, which are vital for longevity, metabolic health, and preventing degeneration.
- Get early warning signals — for example, irregular heart-rate patterns, poor oxygen saturation, or poor recovery — so you can intervene early with lifestyle changes or medical advice.
- Use data-driven insights to adjust diet, exercise, rest and lifestyle for long-term health span enhancement rather than reactive short-term fixes.

In effect wearable health devices can become a personal health coach and tracker that helps you stay consistently aligned with your health and longevity goals. They bring awareness, help you make informed lifestyle decisions, and enable you to proactively manage your health rather than react to problems after they arise.

Chapter 30

Normal Reference Ranges for Key Biomarkers

Following are the normal reference ranges for various important health parameters:

1. Complete Blood Count (CBC)

The CBC evaluates red cells, white cells, and platelets—key indicators of oxygen-carrying capacity, immunity, and blood clotting.

- Haemoglobin: Men 13.8–17.2 g/dL; Women 12.1–15.1 g/dL
- Haematocrit: Men 40.7–50.3%; Women 36.1–44.3%
- RBC Count: Men 4.7–6.1 million/µL; Women 4.2–5.4 million/µL
- WBC Count: 4,500–11,000 cells/µL
- Platelet Count: 150,000–450,000 cells/µL

2. Comprehensive Metabolic Panel (CMP)

This panel reflects electrolyte balance, kidney and liver function, and overall metabolic health.

Electrolytes

- Sodium: 135–145 mmol/L
- Potassium: 3.5–5.1 mmol/L
- Chloride: 98–107 mmol/L
- Calcium: 8.5–10.2 mg/dL
- Magnesium: 1.7–2.2 mg/dL
- Phosphorus: 2.5–4.5 mg/dL

Kidney Markers

- BUN: 7–20 mg/dL
- Creatinine: Men 0.7–1.3 mg/dL; Women 0.6–1.1 mg/dL
- eGFR: >60 mL/min/1.73 m^2
- Uric Acid: Men 3.4–7.0 mg/dL; Women 2.4–6.0 mg/dL

Liver Function

- ALT: 7–56 U/L
- AST: 10–40 U/L
- ALP: 30–120 U/L
- Total Bilirubin: 0.1–1.2 mg/dL
- Albumin: 3.5–5.0 g/dL
- Total Protein: 6.0–8.3 g/dL

Glucose Regulation

- Fasting Glucose: 70–100 mg/dL

3. Lipid Profile

-A vital assessment of cardiovascular risk.

- Total Cholesterol: <200 mg/dL
- LDL Cholesterol (Bad): <100 mg/dL
- HDL Cholesterol (Good): Men >40 mg/dL; Women >50 mg/dL
- Triglycerides: <150 mg/dL

4. Vitamins and Minerals

These reflect nutritional adequacy and metabolic health.

- Vitamin D (25-OH): 30–100 ng/mL
- Vitamin B12: 200–900 pg./mL
- Folate: 2–20 ng/mL

(Other minerals listed earlier under electrolytes.)

5. Blood Sugar and Insulin Markers

-Crucial for diagnosing and monitoring diabetes.

- Fasting Blood Glucose: 70–100 mg/dL
- HbA1c:
    - Normal: <6%
    - Pre-diabetes: 5.7–6.4%
    - Diabetes: ≥6.5%
- Fasting Insulin: 2–25 µU/mL
    - Optimal: 3–6 µU/mL

6. Inflammation and Autoimmune Markers

-Useful for detecting hidden inflammation and autoimmune disorders.

- hs-CRP:
    - <1 mg/L (Low risk)
    - 1–3 mg/L (Moderate)
    - 3 mg/L (High)
- ESR: Men 0–15 mm/hr; Women 0–20 mm/hr
- Rheumatoid Factor (RF): <14 IU/mL
- Anti-CCP Antibodies: <20 U/mL

7. Thyroid Function Tests

Indicate metabolic rate and thyroid health.

- TSH: 0.5–4.5 μIU/mL
- Free T3: 2.3–4.2 pg./mL
- Free T4: 0.8–1.8 ng/dL
- Anti-TPO Antibodies: <35 IU/mL

8. Iron Status and Nutritional Markers

These help confirm iron deficiency, anaemia risk, and nutritional health.

- Serum Iron: 60–170 μg/dL
- Ferritin: Men 24–336 ng/mL; Women 11–307 ng/mL
- TIBC (Total Iron-Binding Capacity): 250–450 μg/dL

9. Cancer Screening Biomarkers

Used selectively for high-risk groups or clinical suspicion.

- PSA (Men): <4.0 ng/mL
- CA-125 (Women): <35 U/mL
- CEA:
    - <5.0 ng/mL for non-smokers
    - <10 ng/mL for smokers

10. Special Considerations for Adults Over 70

Targets shift with age to balance risks—especially hypoglycemia.

- Fasting Blood Sugar:
    - 80–130 mg/dL for healthy older adults
    - 100–150 mg/dL for frail elderly
- HbA1c Goals:

- <7% for healthy individuals
- <7.5–8% when other illnesses are present

- Note: Low blood sugar is more dangerous in the elderly than mildly elevated glucose.

11. Additional Tests Recommended Based on Health Status

General Health Monitoring

- hs-CRP and ESR (inflammation)
- Fasting Insulin (metabolic health)
- PSA for men
- Watch for:
  - Low Sodium (<135 mmol/L)
  - Low Albumin (<3.5 g/dL)
  - Low Total Protein (<6 g/dL)

Longevity and Physical Fitness Assessments

- BOLT (Body Oxygen Level Test)
- Grip Strength Test
- Balance Assessment
- CT Coronary Angiography (non-invasive evaluation for heart blockages)

Chapter 31

Harmony of Yoga with Modern Science

Modern science is increasingly recognizing and validating the ancient wisdom of yoga and pranayama as powerful tools for preventive healthcare. Scientific studies now clearly show physiological and psychological benefits of these practices.

Stress and Heart Health: Consistent practice of yoga and pranayama helps to lower stress hormones like cortisol, reduce blood pressure, and slow the heart rate—all of which support overall cardiovascular health.

Chronic Conditions: Research has linked these practices to improvements in various chronic conditions. Studies show positive effects on managing hypertension, asthma, and diabetes, often by improving lung function, enhancing insulin sensitivity, and reducing systemic inflammation.

Brain and Immunity: The mindful breathing techniques of pranayama, in particular, have been found to directly affect the nervous system, boosting immunity and dramatically improving mental clarity and focus. This scientific validation has led to the growing acceptance of yoga and pranayama as valuable, cost-effective, and holistic tools for disease prevention and maintaining long-term physical and mental health.

Chapter 32

Longevity, Vitality & Happiness

A truly successful life is measured not just by its length, but by its quality. Longevity, Vitality, and Happiness are deeply interconnected elements that influence and complement each other.

Longevity (Lifespan)

Longevity refers to the actual length of a person's life. While genetics play a role, lifestyle choices are far more influential.

Physiological Resilience (the body's ability to recover from stress or disease) naturally declines with age.

A healthy diet, regular exercise, adequate sleep, and avoiding harmful habits (like smoking and excessive alcohol) can significantly slow this decline, extending not just the lifespan but, more importantly, the health span (the years spent in good health).

Vitality (Energy and Health Span)

Vitality is the feeling of being alive and full of energy—physically, mentally, and emotionally. Key factors that enhance vitality include:

Regular Exercise: A balanced mix of cardio and strength training improves mood, boosts energy, and enhances cognitive function by releasing endorphins.

Balanced Nutrition and Hydration: A diet rich in proteins and healthy fats, along with proper hydration, fuels optimal body and brain performance.

Mind-Body Harmony: Consistent practices like yoga and pranayama help balance physical tension and mental stress.
Mental Engagement: Lifelong learning, problem-solving, and social interaction help maintain cognitive function and a sense of fulfilment.

Happiness (Well-being and Resilience)

Happiness is a state of overall well-being, deeply rooted in how we connect with others and how we find meaning in life.
Social Bonds: Strong relationships and positive interactions release feel-good hormones like oxytocin, which reduce stress and strengthen emotional resilience.
Sense of Purpose: Whether achieved through work, volunteering, or hobbies, having a clear purpose gives life direction and meaning.
Daily Joys: Simple acts like expressing gratitude, performing kindness, and practicing mindfulness have been shown to elevate mood and increase life satisfaction.
Happier individuals not only report a better quality of life but also tend to live longer and enjoy better physical health. The mind-body connection is powerful—happiness acts as a catalyst for a longer, more vibrant life.
A truly vibrant life is not just about living longer; it is about living well, with energy, purpose, and joy.

Section 2

How to choose the Right Foods

Chapter 33

Protein: The Key to a Stronger Body

Protein is an essential macronutrient made of building blocks called amino acids. It plays a crucial role in nearly every bodily process, from building and repairing tissues to producing hormones and enzymes. Getting enough protein is the key to:

- Promoting muscle growth, repair, and maintenance.
- Supporting your immune system.
- Aiding in brain function and cognitive health.

How Much Protein Do You Need Daily?

The general recommendation is 1 to 1.5 grams of protein per kilogram of body weight. However, your specific needs can vary based on your age, gender, activity level, and health goals. For example, athletes and people looking to build muscle may need more protein than the average sedentary person.

Top Protein Sources

You can easily meet your daily protein needs by including a variety of high-protein foods in your diet.

High-Protein Non-Vegetarian Foods (per 100g cooked)

Food Item	Protein (per 100g cooked)
Chicken Breast (skinless)	31 g
Pork (lean)	27 g
Beef (lean)	26–28 g
Mutton/Lamb	25–27 g
Prawns (cooked)	24 g
Fish – Surmai (Kingfish/Seer)	25–27 g
Fish – Rawas (Indian Salmon)	22–25 g
Fish – Bangda (Mackerel)	20–22 g
Fish – Rohu (Carp)	17–20 g
Egg (1 medium, ~50g)	6.5–7 g

High-Protein Vegetarian Foods (per 100g cooked)

Food Item	Protein (per 100g cooked)
Soybeans	16.6 g
Chickpeas (chana)	8.9 g
Split Chickpeas (Chana dal)	8.8 g
Kidney Beans (Rajma)	8.7 g
Split Red Lentils (Masoor dal)	7.6 g
Moth Beans (Matki)	7.6 g
Split Pigeon Pea (Tur dal)	7.2 g
Split Green Gram (Moong dal)	7.0 g
Green Gram (Moong)	7.0 g
Oats	2.6 g

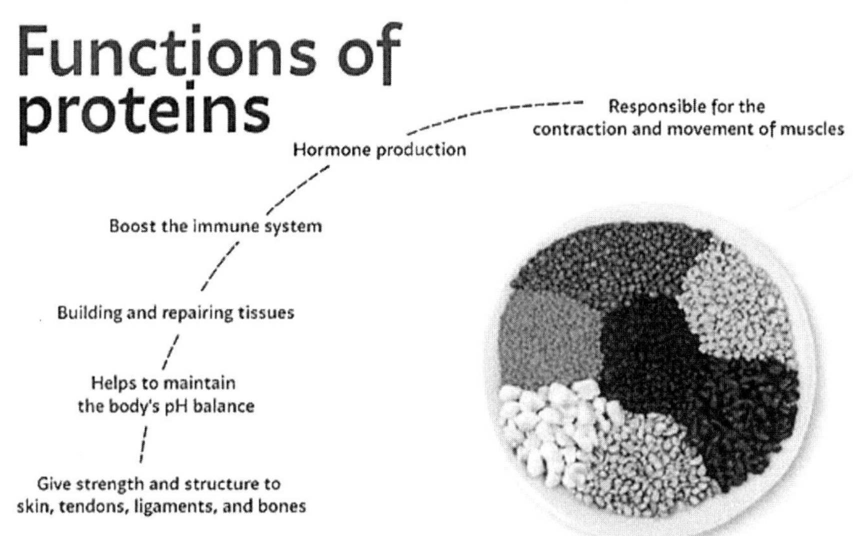

Amazing high protein foods

There are some extraordinary animal-based and plant-based foods with high protcin content. One can easily achieve the daily requirement of proteins by consuming them.

Food Item	Approximate Protein (per 100g)
Soya Granules / Flakes (Dry)	50-54 g
Fish (cooked, e.g., Salmon, Tuna)	20-26 g
Chicken Breast (cooked, skinless)	30-32 g
Skinless Chicken Drumsticks (cooked)	20-25 g
Egg Whites (raw)	11 g
Cottage Cheese (Paneer)	18-20 g
Chia Seeds	17 g
Flax Seeds	18 g
Almonds	21 g
Peanuts	24-26 g

Food Item	Approximate Protein (per 100g)
Walnuts	15 g

Importance of Leucine

Leucine is a component of protein. It is an Essential Amino Acid. Leucine is particularly important because it has a special role beyond just being a building block. It activates Muscle Growth. It acts as a powerful signal that turns on the cellular pathway responsible for muscle protein synthesis (mTOR pathway). This makes it crucial for muscle repair and growth.

Whey Protein, Pumpkin seeds, Almonds and Peanuts have a high concentration of Leucine and hence you should plan to include these in breakfast.

Understanding Whey Protein

Whey is a natural component of milk that is separated as a liquid byproduct during the process of converting milk into curd. It is produced on large scale during cheese production. It is a high-quality protein valued for its rich profile of essential amino acids and rapid absorption.

A good quality whey protein supplement contains about 80% protein.

Whey protein is particularly beneficial for older adults. It can help prevent age-related muscle loss and supports bone health due to its high protein and calcium content.

Whey protein concentrate is scientifically considered the highest quality protein due to its superior Biological Value meaning the body uses it incredibly efficiently. It has a high concentration of Leucine, which is the primary trigger for muscle protein synthesis. It is digested and absorbed quickly, making it ideal for muscle repair and recovery.

Best Ways to Consume Whey Protein:

Smoothies: Blend with milk or water, fruits, and nuts.

Soups & Dals: Stir into soups or cooked dal after removing from the stove.

Breakfast: Add to oatmeal or porridge.

Fermented Drinks: Mix with buttermilk or curd for easy digestion.

Most whey protein brands are available in 1kg containers with a 30 ml scoop. A common dosage is one scoop per day, which provides around 24 grams of protein.

Learning

Proteins are large, complex molecules made up of chains of smaller units called amino acids, which are often referred to as the body's building blocks. While the body can synthesize many amino acids, nine are considered essential amino acids and must be obtained through the diet. Protein is a power packed nutrient vital for a stronger, healthier body. By ensuring that you get enough protein from a variety of sources—whether plant or animal-based—you can significantly enhance your physical health and well-being.

Chapter 34

Fats & Cooking Oils –Good, Bad & Acceptable

Fats are essential macronutrients that serve as a major source of energy for the body. Found in both plant and animal foods, dietary fats support cell growth, protect organs, help absorb vitamins (A, D, E, and K), and aid in hormone production. Our body also makes fat by converting excess calories into stored fat. Fats are essential for good health. They power the body, support the brain, protect organs, balance hormones, and improve heart health when consumed wisely.

Importance of Fats

Fats are essential macronutrient that plays a vital role in keeping the body healthy. Although often misunderstood, the right fats are crucial for energy, hormones, brain function, and overall well-being. Rather than avoiding fats completely, it is important to choose the right type and consume them in balanced amounts.

1. Provide Concentrated Energy

Fats are the body's most energy-dense nutrient, supplying more than double the calories of carbohydrates or proteins. They act as a long-lasting fuel source, especially during fasting, endurance activities, or when energy demand is high.

2. Support Cell Structure and Brain Health

Every cell membrane in the body is made up of fat. Healthy fats—especially omega-3 fatty acids—are essential for brain development, memory, mood regulation, and nerve function. Nearly 60% of the brain is fat, making the quality of dietary fat highly important.

3. Help Absorb Vitamins

Fat enables the absorption of fat-soluble vitamins A, D, E, and K, which are vital for immunity, bone health, vision, blood clotting, and antioxidant protection. Without adequate dietary fat, these vitamins cannot be absorbed properly.

4. Essential for Hormone Production

Many hormones—including those regulating metabolism, stress, mood, and reproduction—require fats for their synthesis. Healthy fats help maintain hormonal balance throughout life.

5. Protect Organs and Regulate Body Temperature

Fats cushion vital organs, protect against impact, and help maintain body temperature. The fat layer under the skin acts as natural insulation.

6. Healthy Fats Reduce Inflammation and Support Heart Health

Unsaturated fats found in nuts, seeds, olive oil, avocados, and fatty fish help reduce inflammation, improve cholesterol levels, lower blood pressure, and protect the heart. Omega-3 fats, in particular, are strongly linked to reduced risk of cardiovascular disease.

However, all fats are not created equal and they have different effect on health. Understanding the different types of fats and their impact on health is important for choosing the right type.

1. The Only Healthy Fats – Unsaturated Fats

Unsaturated fats are the stars among fats. They are heart-friendly, remain liquid at room temperature, and come mainly from plant sources and fish.

They help reduce bad cholesterol (LDL), increase good cholesterol (HDL), and protect against heart disease.

Types of Healthy Fats:

A. Monounsaturated Fats (MUFA)

Found in:

- Olive oil, peanut oil, sunflower oil, mustard oil, rice bran oil, safflower oil, and corn oil
- Avocados, almonds, peanuts, and other nuts and seeds

Foods Rich in Monounsaturated Fats (per 100 g)

Food Item	MUFA (g)
Olive oil	73
Canola oil	62
Peanut oil	46
Hazelnuts	46
Almonds	32
Sunflower oil	70–80
Avocado	30
Pecans	40
Pistachios	24

Food Item	MUFA (g)
Peanuts	24
Sesame oil	40
Dark chocolate	25–30

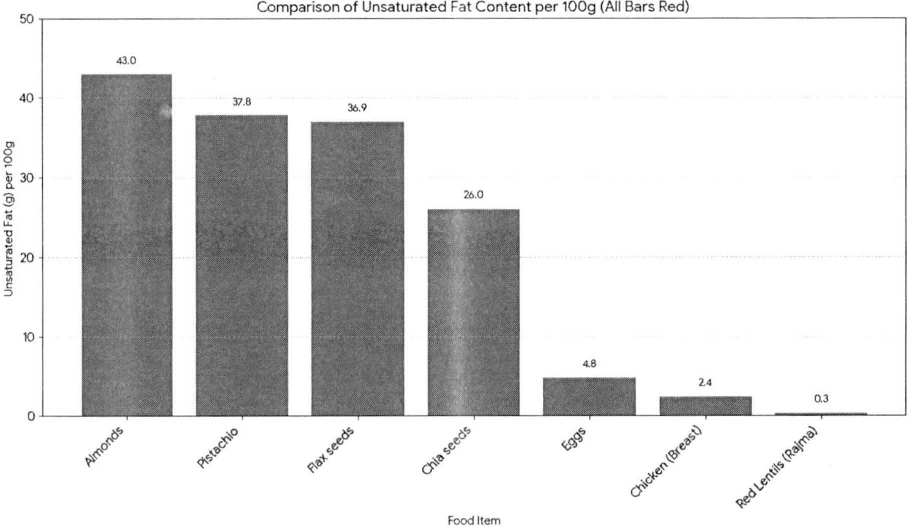

B. Polyunsaturated Fats (PUFA)

Also known as Omega-3 and Omega-6 Fatty Acids, these are essential fats that our body cannot produce and must be obtained from food. Found in:

- Vegetable oils like soybean, sunflower, safflower, corn, and canola oil
- Nuts and seeds such as flaxseeds, chia seeds, walnuts, almonds, and sunflower seeds
- Oily fish like salmon, tuna, sardine, herring, mackerel, rohu, rawas, surmai, pomfret, and katla

Foods Rich in Polyunsaturated Fats (per 100 g)

Food Item	PUFA (g)
Flaxseed oil	66
Safflower oil	75
Sunflower oil	65
Corn oil	59
Soybean oil	58
Chia seeds	31
Flaxseeds	42
Hemp seeds	28
Pumpkin seeds	20
Walnuts	47
Indian fatty fish (Surmai, Rohu, Rawas, Pomfret)	5–10
Salmon, Mackerel, Sardine, Herring	~10

Omega-3: Essential Fats for Optimal Health

Omega-3 fatty acids are a family of polyunsaturated healthy fats that are absolutely essential for human health. Because the body can't produce them on its own, they must be obtained through diet, classifying them as essential fatty acids (EFAs). These fats are vital for the heart, brain, and overall inflammation management.

There are three primary forms of omega-3s that are important in human nutrition:

1. EPA: Known for its powerful anti-inflammatory properties and its direct benefits to cardiovascular health.
2. DHA: A crucial structural component of the brain, retina, and cell membranes. It is especially vital for brain development and function throughout life.

3. ALA: This is the plant-based precursor. The body must convert ALA into the more active forms, EPA and DHA, but this conversion process is typically inefficient (often less than 10%).

The extensive research on omega-3s highlights their profound impact on various body systems:

Omega-3s can significantly reduce several risk factors for heart disease. They are known to lower high triglycerides, slightly reduce blood pressure, decrease inflammation, and prevent abnormal heart rhythms.

DHA makes up a large percentage of the fat in the brain. Adequate intake is linked to better cognitive function across all ages and may help manage symptoms of depression and anxiety.

DHA is highly concentrated in the retina of the eye. It is thought to play a role in reducing the risk of macular degeneration.

Omega-3s help balance the body's inflammatory response, which is crucial since chronic, low-grade inflammation is a driver of many diseases, including arthritis and autoimmune conditions.

To ensure you get enough of these beneficial fats, it's important to include both animal and plant sources in your diet. Examples are:

Fatty Fish like Salmon, mackerel, sardines, herring, anchovies, Flaxseeds, Chia Seeds, Walnuts and Soybean

2. The Most Harmful Fats – Trans Fats

Trans fats are the villains of the fat world. Most are industrially produced by hydrogenation, a process that turns cheap liquid oils (palm, soybean, corn) into solid fats to extend shelf life and improve texture in processed foods.

Why Trans Fats Are Harmful

1. Raise bad cholesterol (LDL) and lower good cholesterol (HDL)
2. Increase risk of heart disease, stroke, and type 2 diabetes
3. Promote inflammation and insulin resistance

Common sources:

- Packaged baked goods (cakes, cookies, pastries, muffins)
- Fried fast food (doughnuts, French fries)
- Frozen pizzas, crackers, and processed snacks

Many countries, including the US and UK, have banned trans fats, but they still sneak into diets through imported products and unregulated local markets.

3. Just Acceptable Fats – Saturated Fats

Saturated fats fall into a grey zone—neither completely good nor entirely bad.

They are usually solid at room temperature and should be consumed in moderation, as excess intake raises LDL cholesterol and increases the risk of heart disease.

Common Sources:

- Red meat (beef, pork, lamb) and poultry with skin
- Full-fat dairy products (milk, cheese, butter, ghee)
- Coconut oil and palm oil
- Pizza, cheese, and bakery products made with butter or shortening

Foods High in Saturated Fat (per 100 g)

Food Item	Saturated Fat (g)
Coconut oil	82
Ghee (clarified butter)	62
Butter	51
Palm oil	50
Heavy cream	23
Cheese (Cheddar, etc.)	19–21
Milk/white chocolate	12–19
Processed meats (sausages, salami)	9–15
Fatty red meat (beef, lamb, pork)	7–13
Baked goods (cakes, pastries, cookies)	8–20

Recommended Limit

-WHO and American Heart Association recommend that consumption of Saturated fats should be restricted to less than 5–8% of total daily calories. In practical terms this works out to about 10–15 g per day.

Saturated Fat content in popular foods:

- 1 tbsp ghee -9 g
- 100 g paneer (full-fat) -14 g
- 1 cup whole milk -5 g
- 100 g coconut oil - 82 g (very high!)

It is better to replace butter and ghee with olive oil, mustard oil, or canola oil. Also, include nuts, seeds, avocados, and fatty fish for healthier eating.

COOKING OILS – CHOOSING THE RIGHT ONE

The choice of cooking oil depends on taste, heat stability (smoke point), and type of cooking.

Common Oils in the Western countries

- Canola, Sunflower, and Peanut oil – Neutral flavor, suitable for frying and general cooking
- Olive oil – Used widely in Mediterranean cooking for roasting, sautéing, and dressing
  Extra Virgin Olive Oil: For low-heat cooking and salads
  Regular Olive Oil: For everyday cooking
- Corn and Soybean oils – Often used in blended "vegetable oils" for frying

Common Oils in India

Indian cooking demands oils that tolerate high heat and match regional flavours.

Cooking Method	**Best Oils**	**Notes**
Sautéing (vegetables, curry base)	Mustard, Groundnut, Sunflower	Medium–high heat, minimal oil
Shallow Frying (cutlets, parathas, fish fry)	Groundnut, Mustard, Sesame, Coconut	Crisp texture, medium–high heat
Stir-Frying (Indo-Chinese, quick veg/non-veg)	Groundnut, Sesame	Very high heat, little oil

Cooking Method	Best Oils	Notes
Deep Frying (pakoras, samosas, puris)	Groundnut, Mustard, Sunflower	High heat, large oil quantity
Oils for General Cooking: – *Sunflower oil*: North/Central India; mild flavor for daily use – *Groundnut oil*: Maharashtra, Gujarat; good for frying, tadka – *Mustard oil*: Bengal, Punjab, Bihar, UP; gives depth to curries – *Coconut oil*: Kerala, coastal Karnataka; ideal for seafood, curries – *Sesame oil (Til)*: Tamil Nadu; adds aroma to chutneys, pickles – *Ghee*: Used across India for dal tadka, rajma, finishing dishes		

Golden Rules for Using Oils

- Use less oil whenever possible
- Rotate oils (e.g., mustard, groundnut, sesame, coconut) instead of sticking to one type
- Avoid reusing oil for frying – reheating forms harmful compounds
- Prefer cold-pressed oils for low-heat cooking
- Reserve deep-frying for occasional treats – sautéing should be your everyday method

Learning:

Fats are classified into three main types: Saturated, Unsaturated and Trans fats. Unsaturated fats, particularly those high in Omega-3 and Omega-6 fatty acids, are considered the healthiest choice as they support heart and brain health and help lower bad cholesterol (LDL). Saturated fats, often solid at room temperature, should be consumed in moderation, while artificial trans fats, which raise LDL and lower good cholesterol (HDL), should be strictly avoided. The key to a healthy diet is replacing saturated and trans fats with beneficial unsaturated fats from sources like fish, nuts, seeds, and vegetable oils.

Chapter 35

Fibrous Foods – Say Goodbye to Constipation

Dietary fibre, often overlooked, is absolutely necessary in every healthy diet. It's a powerful agent in combating constipation and offers several additional health benefits.

What is Dietary Fiber?

It is the indigestible part of plant-based foods. It passes through the digestive system largely intact and is classified into two broad categories based on water solubility:

Soluble fibre: Dissolves in water, forming a gel-like substance. It can help lower blood cholesterol and regulate blood sugar.

Insoluble fibre: Does not dissolve in water. It adds bulk to the stool and helps food pass more quickly through the stomach and intestines.

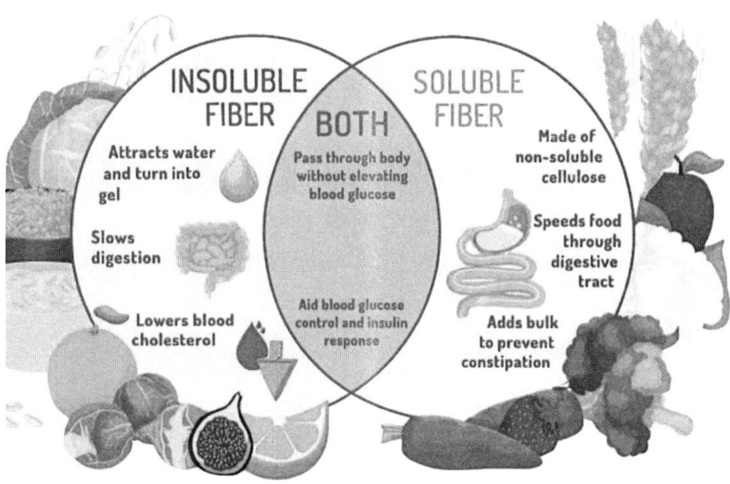

Why Is Fiber Important?

1. Promotes Healthy Digestion and Prevents Constipation.

Insoluble fibre increases stool bulk and speeds up intestinal movement, effectively preventing and relieving constipation. Soluble fibre absorbs water and softens the stool, making it easier to pass.

2. Supports Gut Microbiome

The gut hosts trillions of beneficial bacteria. These bacteria help regulate immune function, mood, metabolism, and more. Fiber acts as a prebiotic, feeding these "good" bacteria and supporting a healthy microbiome.

3. Helps Control Blood Sugar Levels

Soluble fibre slows the absorption of sugar, reducing blood sugar spikes after meals and improving glycaemic control, particularly important for people with diabetes.

4. Aids in Weight Management

Fiber increases satiety, helping you feel fuller for longer, which can lead to reduced calorie intake and better weight control.

5. May Reduce Risk of Heart Disease

Fiber, especially from whole plant foods, has been linked to lower levels of LDL (bad) cholesterol.

What is Daily Fiber requirement?

Health authorities recommend the following daily intake of dietary fibre:

Adult men: 38 grams

Adult women: 25 grams

Best Sources of Dietary Fiber

To reap the full benefits of fibre, a variety of foods should be included in your diet. Here are some excellent high-fibre foods, organized by category:

Fruits (one medium fruit):

Raspberries – 8 g, Pear – 5.5 g, Apple – 4.5 g, Banana-3 g

Orange – 3 g, Strawberries – 3 g

Vegetables (per 1 cup):

Green peas, boiled – 9 g, Broccoli, boiled – 5 g, Turnip greens – 5 g, Brussels sprouts – 4.5 g, Potato – 4 g, sweet corn – 4 g

Grains and Cereals (per 1 cup):

Whole-wheat spaghetti – 6 g, Barley – 6 g, Quinoa – 5 g

Oatmeal – 4 g, Brown rice – 3.5 g

Legumes, Nuts, and Seeds:

Split peas – 16 g, Lentils – 15.5 g, Black beans – 15, Chickpeas – 8 g (per ½ cup), Chia seeds – 10 g (per ounce) Almonds – 3.5 g (per ounce), Pistachios – 3 g (per ounce)

How Insoluble Fiber Prevents Constipation

Insoluble fibre acts as a natural laxative. As it travels through your digestive system, it absorbs water and increases the bulk of your stool. This bulkier stool stimulates the intestinal walls to contract more effectively, moving waste through your colon faster. This prevents the stool from becoming hard and dry, which is a common cause of constipation. Insoluble fibre, thus acts as a natural laxative, encouraging regularity without the need for medication.

Learning

Though not a nutrient in the conventional sense, dietary fibre plays an essential role in maintaining health. It supports digestion, blood sugar regulation, and gut microbiome balance. Including a wide variety of fruits, vegetables, legumes, nuts, seeds, and whole grains in your diet can ensure a rich and beneficial intake of dietary fibre. Say goodbye to constipation and hello to a healthier, more comfortable life.

Chapter 36

Vitamins & Minerals Your Body Needs

In order to appreciate the value of vitamins truly, we must first understand the role of free radicals and antioxidants. Free radicals are unstable molecules generated during the conversion of food into energy. They can also enter the body through pollutants, processed foods, and tobacco smoke. These highly reactive molecules can damage cells, accelerate aging, and contribute to chronic diseases.

Vitamins protect the body by neutralizing free radicals. This antioxidant action supports cellular health and helps the body resist disease and deterioration.

Why Are Vitamins Essential?

Vitamins are essential micronutrients required for numerous physiological processes. They support immune health, promote energy production, assist in cell growth and repair, and regulate metabolism. Since the human body cannot produce most vitamins or produces some in small quantities, they must be obtained through diet or supplements.

Important Vitamins and Their Food Sources

Vitamin A: Vital for vision, immune defence, and skin health. Found in carrots, sweet potatoes, spinach, and dairy products.

Vitamin B Complex: A group of eight vitamins that support brain function, red blood cell production, and energy metabolism. Found in whole grains, meat, eggs, legumes, and dairy.

Vitamin C – Strengthens immunity, enhances collagen synthesis, and acts as a powerful antioxidant. Found in citrus fruits, strawberries, bell peppers, and tomatoes.
Vitamin D – Aids in calcium absorption and supports bone and immune health. It is obtained through sunlight exposure, fortified dairy, fatty fish, and egg yolks.
Vitamin E – Protects cells from damage by free radicals and supports immune response. Found in nuts, seeds, vegetable oils, and leafy greens.
Vitamin K – Essential for blood clotting and bone metabolism. Found in leafy greens like kale and spinach, and fermented foods.

Role of Vitamin D & Vitamin B12 During Sleep

Although neither Vitamin D nor Vitamin B12 directly induces sleep, both are essential for the quality of sleep, maintenance of the biological clock, night-time repair, and regulation of key hormones and neural pathways that operate most actively during sleep.

Role of Vitamin D:

- Regulates Sleep–Wake Rhythm

Vitamin D receptors exist in brain regions controlling sleep. Supports stable circadian rhythms and melatonin signalling. Low levels are linked to insomnia, shorter sleep, and more awakenings.

- Boosts Immune Repair at Night

-Enhances T-cell activation and immune defence.
-Reduces systemic inflammation, which otherwise disrupts sleep.
-Supports the body's night-time healing cycles.

- Supports Muscle and Bone Recovery

-Facilitates calcium metabolism during deep sleep.

Enhances muscle repair and bone remodelling.

Helps reduce night cramps and restless sleep.

Role of Vitamin B12:

- Maintains the Internal Body Clock

Helps synchronise circadian rhythm and sleep timing.

Important for morning alertness and consistent sleep schedules.

- Aids Melatonin Pathway (Indirectly)

Supports conversion of tryptophan to serotonin, later converted to melatonin.

-Promotes smoother sleep onset and stable night-time rhythm.

- Supports Nervous System Repair

-Essential for myelin maintenance and nerve regeneration during deep sleep. Low levels contribute to restless legs, vivid dreams, and fragmented sleep. Helps maintain neurotransmitter balance for calmer sleep.

- Lowers Night-time Homocysteine

High homocysteine impairs blood vessels and disrupts restorative sleep. B12 actively reduces homocysteine during overnight metabolic cycles.

Recommended Daily Intake

- Vitamin C: 200 to 400 mg/day
- Vitamin D3: 1000 to 2000 IU /day
- Vitamin B12: 250 to 500 mcg/day

Comparison of Vitamin C, Vitamin D, and Vitamin B12

Vitamin C, Vitamin D, and Vitamin B12 are three essential vitamins that play very different roles in the body. Together, they support energy, immunity, sleep quality, metabolism, and long-term health.

- Vitamin C is a water-soluble antioxidant that works throughout the day to neutralise free radicals. It strengthens the immune system, accelerates wound healing, improves iron absorption, supports collagen formation, and protects blood vessels. Because it is not stored, it must be taken regularly through diet. It is found in Citrus fruits, amla, guava, kiwi, berries, tomatoes, and bell peppers.

- Vitamin D is a fat-soluble vitamin, produced when sunlight hits the skin. It regulates calcium, bone strength, muscle function, immune activity, and inflammatory balance. It also interacts with brain regions that control sleep and circadian rhythm. It is found in Sunlight, fortified milk, eggs, mushrooms, but dietary sources alone seldom meet requirements

- Vitamin B12 is a water-soluble vitamin essential for the nervous system. It maintains the myelin sheath around nerves, supports memory and concentration, reduces homocysteine, and is vital for DNA synthesis and red blood cell production. Absorption decreases with age and is low in vegetarian diets, making supplementation common. It is found in Milk, curd, paneer, cheese, eggs, fish, and fortified cereals. Plant foods do not contain B12.

Symptoms of Deficiency

Vitamin C deficiency causes fatigue, low immunity, slow wound healing, gum bleeding, easy bruising, and rough skin.

Vitamin D deficiency causes tiredness, bone pain, muscle weakness, low immunity, mood changes, poor sleep, and long-term risk of osteoporosis.

Vitamin B12 deficiency causes tingling in hands/feet, fatigue, poor memory, mood changes, restless legs, imbalance, and anaemia. Even mild deficiency affects sleep quality and nerve function.

Why Are Minerals Important?

Minerals are inorganic elements crucial for maintaining health. They support bone and muscle strength, nerve transmission, hormone production, and fluid balance. Though required in smaller quantities, their absence can lead to serious health complications.

Role of key Minerals

Calcium – Builds and maintains bones and teeth. Aids in blood clotting, nerve function, and muscle contraction.

Magnesium – Regulates muscle and nerve activity, blood pressure, and supports DNA and protein synthesis.

Zinc – Essential for immune function, wound healing, and enzyme activity. Also important for taste and smell.

Iron – Enables red blood cells to transport oxygen. Prevents anaemia and supports energy levels.

Potassium – Balances body fluids, maintains normal blood pressure, and supports nerve and muscle function.

Why Magnesium is needed?

Magnesium is vital for muscle relaxation, sleep quality, and anxiety reduction. It helps maintain a steady heartbeat, regulates blood pressure, and supports bone health when combined with calcium and vitamin D. Deficiency symptoms include muscle cramps, irritability, fatigue, and insomnia.

Why Zinc is needed?

Zinc boosts immune defence, facilitates wound healing, and supports DNA synthesis. Deficiency can lead to reduced immunity, skin disorders, hair thinning, and diminished taste and smell.

Why Vitamin B12 is needed?

Vitamin B12 is essential for red blood cell formation, neurological function, and DNA production. As people age, their ability to absorb B12 decreases, making supplementation important to prevent fatigue, memory issues, and nerve damage.

Important Supplements to Consider

Vitamin D3:

-Supports immune function, bone health, and mood regulation

-Especially important for those with limited sun exposure

Magnesium Glycinate:

-Aids sleep, muscle function, and cardiovascular health

Omega-3 Fatty Acids (EPA & DHA):

-Promote brain health, reduce inflammation, and support heart function

-Commonly sourced from fish oil or algae-based supplements

-Enhances cognitive performance and muscle energy

-Beneficial not only for athletes but also for aging and brain health

Vitamin K2:

-Works synergistically with Vitamin D for bone and cardiovascular health

-Helps direct calcium to bones and away from arteries

Learning:

Vitamins are classified as fat-soluble (A, D, E, K), which are stored in the body's fatty tissues, and water-soluble (C and all B vitamins), which are not stored and must be consumed regularly. Minerals are inorganic elements vital for building strong bones and teeth (like Calcium), carrying oxygen in the blood (Iron), maintaining fluid balance (Sodium, Potassium), and supporting nerve and muscle function. Both micronutrients, though required in tiny quantities, are critical; a deficiency in either can lead to specific diseases, highlighting the importance of a varied, nutrient-dense diet.

Chapter 37

Eggs, Curd, and Paneer- Nutritional Powerhouse

Eggs

Eggs are an excellent source of high-quality protein and healthy fats. The protein in eggs has the highest biological value, meaning it contains all the essential amino acids your body needs. For this reason, it is considered the "gold standard" for evaluating protein in other foods.

A large egg (50g) contains about 6 grams of protein (4g in the white, 2g in the yolk), 5g of fat, and 60 calories.

Eggs are also rich in minerals like iodine, zinc, selenium, and iron.

Is Egg yolk good or bad?

While egg yolks contain cholesterol, recent research shows that for most healthy people, dietary cholesterol has a minimal impact on blood cholesterol levels. The yolk is a nutrient powerhouse, so for most people, consuming the whole egg is good for a balanced diet.

Milk – The Original Complete Food

Milk is often called a "complete food" due to its rich content of protein, fat, carbohydrates, vitamins, and minerals.

Milk is a rich source of Protein, Calcium and Vitamin B12

250 ml milk has 8 gm of protein, 8 gm of Fat and approx. 130 calories

It contains 300 mg of Calcium and 1.2 micrograms of Vit B 12.

Milk is easy to digest and helps boost immunity and support healthy growth, especially in children.

Yogurt (Curd) – Your Daily Dose of Good Bacteria

Curd (or yogurt) is more than just fermented milk; it is a probiotic-rich powerhouse that enhances digestion and supports overall gut health. One litre of milk makes 1 litre of curd.

Micronutrients in Curd (per 100 g made from cow milk)

-Protein: 3.5–4 g

-Saturated fat: 1.5 g

-Unsaturated fat: 1.0–1.5 g

-Cholesterol: 10–15 mg

-Calories: 60

It also contains the following minerals and vitamins:

-Calcium & Phosphorus – Strengthen bones and teeth

-Vitamin B12 & Riboflavin – Boost energy and brain health

-Vitamin D – Promotes calcium absorption

-Magnesium & Potassium – Regulate blood pressure and nerve function

-Zinc – Enhances immunity and skin health

Curd and Gut Health

A healthy gut is the foundation of overall wellness.

Probiotics in curd:

-Improve digestion & nutrient absorption

-Strengthen immunity

-Reduce acidity and bloating

-Regulate bowel movements

-Boost mood by supporting serotonin production

Paneer – Delicious and Protein-Rich

Paneer (Indian cottage cheese) is a delicious and nutritious product made by curdling milk with lemon juice or vinegar and straining the solids. It takes about 5–6 litres of milk to make 1 kg of paneer.

Micronutrients in Paneer (per 100 g)

Protein: 18 g

Saturated fat: 8–9 g

Unsaturated fat: 7 g

Cholesterol: 55–60 mg

Calories: 260–280 kcal

What Makes Paneer a Star?

Paneer is an incredibly versatile and nutritious food and is a favourite source of protein in many vegetarian diets.

-Protein: A solid 18–20g of protein per 100.

-Healthy Fats: Includes Omega-3 and Omega-6 fatty acids

-Fibre: Helps regulate digestion

-Immunity Booster: Rich in key vitamins and minerals

Learning:

Milk is a highly nutritious liquid food, serving as an excellent source of readily available calcium for bone health, high-quality protein, and several vitamins (like D and B12). Eggs, though not a dairy product, are often grouped with them due to their similar role as a versatile protein source, providing the highest biological value protein along with essential nutrients like choline and lutein. Curd (or yogurt), made by fermenting milk, is rich in probiotics—beneficial bacteria that support gut health. Finally, Paneer is a concentrated source of casein protein and fat, making it a valuable, energy-dense food, particularly for vegetarians. Together, these foods offer a powerful combination of complete proteins, healthy fats, calcium, and various micronutrients vital for a balanced diet.

Chapter 38

Fish- A Magnificent Treasure

Fish is a nutritional powerhouse. Its unique blend of high-quality protein and an extraordinary concentration of omega-3 fatty acids offers wide-ranging benefits, from brain function to heart health. Fish should, therefore, form an indispensable part of a balanced diet.

Why Fish Deserves the Crown

One of the most remarkable aspects of fish is its unmatched concentration of omega-3 fatty acids, particularly EPA and DHA. These polyunsaturated fats are not produced by the human body and must be obtained through diet—making fatty fish an exceptional source of nutrition.

Omega-3s are potent anti-inflammatory agents that help reduce the risk of cardiovascular disease, arthritis, joint inflammation, Cognitive decline and neurodegenerative disorders

Fish provides complete, high-quality protein, containing all nine essential amino acids. Most fish offer 18–25 grams of protein per 100 grams—often outperforming chicken and legumes.

Rich in Essential Vitamins and Minerals

Fish is one of the richest dietary sources of nutrients often lacking in modern diets:

-*Vitamin D*: Supports bone strength, immunity, and mood stability

-*Vitamin B12*: Vital for nerve function and red blood cell formation

-*Iodine*: Crucial for thyroid function and metabolism

-*Selenium*: A powerful antioxidant that protects cells from oxidative stress

-*Zinc*: Supports immune health, wound healing, and DNA repair

Nutritional Comparison: Fish vs. Other Protein Sources

Nutrient (Per 100g)	Fish (e.g., Rohu)	Chicken	Egg	Lentils (Cooked)
Protein	18–22 g	20–22 g	13 g	7–9 g
Omega-3 Fatty Acids	2–3.5 g	0.1 g	0.05 g	Negligible
Saturated Fats	Low	Moderate	Moderate	Negligible
Vitamin D	High	Very Low	Low	None
Vitamin B12	High	Moderate	Moderate	Very Low

Following chart highlights that Fish is an overwhelmingly superior source of Omega-3 Fatty Acids compared to the other foods like Chicken or Lentils or Eggs.

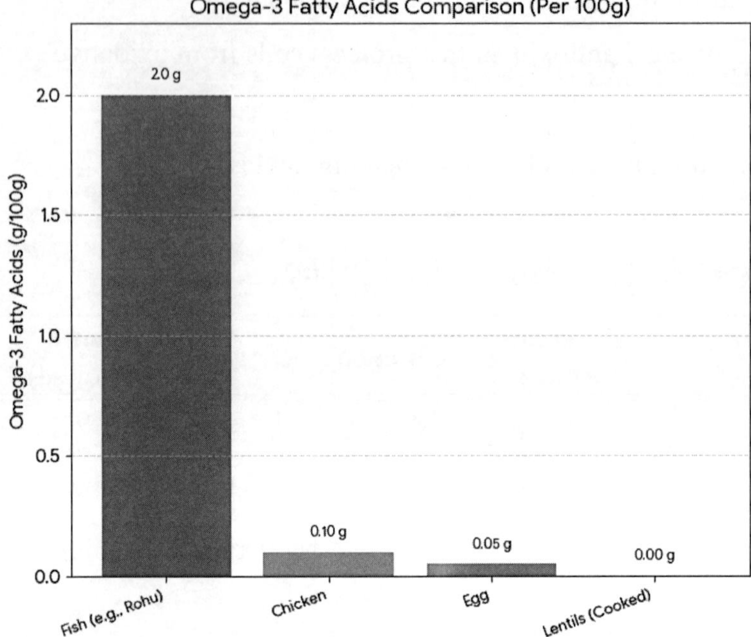

The chart below shows that Fish and Chicken contain almost same amount of protein, much more than Egg or Lentils.

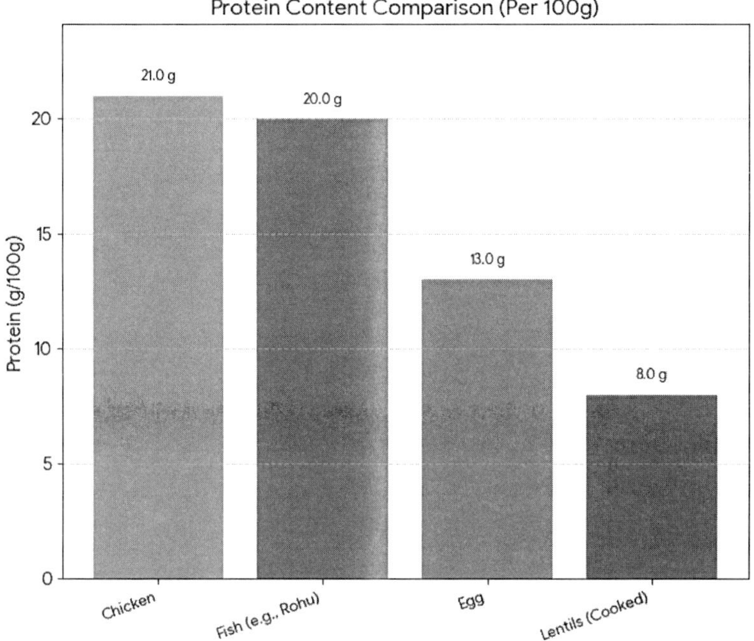

Fish outshines both plant-based and many animal-based proteins by combining lean protein, heart-healthy fats, and a broader micronutrient spectrum. Sardines and Hilsa are among the richest in omega-3. Rawas is considered highly heart-friendly. Pomfret is popular for its mild taste and ease of cooking.

Nutritional Content (per 100g) - Indian Fish

Fish Type	Calories	Protein	Total Fat	Saturated Fat	Unsaturated Fat
Rohu (Rui)	95–97 kcal	17–19g	1.0–2.7g	0.3–2g	0.7–2.4g
Hilsa (Ilish)	222–310 kcal	18–21g	8.2–19.5g	~2–4g	6.2–17.5g
Pomfret (Black)	99–123 kcal	18–20g	2.6–4.8g	0.7–2.2g	1.9–2.6g
Mackerel (Bangda)	189–205 kcal	18–20g	11.9–13.9g	3–3.3g	8.9–10.6g
Indian Salmon (Rawas)	136–203 kcal	20–22g	4.9–13.1g	~1–3g	3.9–10.1g
Surmai (King Mackerel)	105–134 kcal	19–21g	3.3–4.5g	0.9–1.3g	2.4–3.2g

Key Observations:

All these fish are excellent sources of high-quality protein, typically offering 16–22 grams per 100g. Surmai often leads in protein content. Oily fish like Hilsa, Mackerel, and Indian Salmon are rich in both protein and beneficial unsaturated fats. Leaner fish like Rohu and Pomfret still deliver good amount of protein as well as healthy fats.

Top rated Fish in Western countries

- Fatty Fish (Best for Omega-3s)

Salmon: Unquestionably the most popular and highly-rated fish. It is prized for its high content of Omega-3 fatty acids (EPA and DHA), which are excellent for heart and brain health.

Mackerel: A very rich source of Omega-3s and selenium. It's often consumed canned or smoked, especially in European diets.
Sardines and Herring: These small, canned oily fish are highly rated by nutritionists because they are extremely rich in Omega-3s, low in mercury, and high in calcium

- White Fish (Best for Lean Protein)

Cod: Cod is highly consumed and rated for being very lean (low in fat), and an excellent source of high-quality protein and Vitamin B12.
Tuna (Canned Light/Skipjack): Canned tuna is one of the most consumed and most affordable sources of lean protein in the West.
Tilapia: Although often criticized for having fewer Omega-3s than fatty fish, it is one of the most widely consumed due to its mild flavour and low cost.

Nutritional Content (per 100g)-Western Fish

Fish	Protein (g)	Total Fat (g)	Saturated Fat (g)	Unsaturated Fat (g)
Salmon	20–25	10–15	2–3	8–12
Cod	18–20	0.5–1	0.1–0.2	0.4–0.8
Tuna	23–26	1–5	0.2–1	0.8–4
Mackerel	18–20	12–18	3–4	9–14
Haddock	20–22	0.5–1	0.1–0.2	0.4–0.8
Halibut	20–24	2–5	0.5–1	1.5–4
Trout	20–24	5–10	1–2	4–8

Fish	Protein (g)	Total Fat (g)	Saturated Fat (g)	Unsaturated Fat (g)
Herring	18–20	12–18	2.5–4	9–14
Sardines	20–25	10–15	2–3	8–12

Key Observations:

Oily fish (Salmon, Mackerel, Trout, Herring, Sardines) are rich in omega-3s and support heart, brain, and joint health. Lean white fish (Cod, Haddock) offer excellent protein with minimal saturated fat, though omega-3 content is lower.

Comparison of top Indian Fish- Rawas, Surmai, and Rohu:

1. Rawas (Indian Salmon)
   - Protein Content: Very High (approx. 22–26g per 100g).
   - Omega-3 Content: Highest (approx. 1000–2260 mg per 100g).
   - Ranking: #1 for Omega-3 content, making it excellent for heart and brain health. Its high-fat content (healthy fats) is responsible for this superior Omega-3 level.
2. Surmai (Seer Fish)
   - Protein Content: Highest (approx. 20–26g per 100g).
   - Omega-3 Content: High (approx. 400–1200 mg per 100g).
   - Ranking: #1 for Protein among the three, as it is a very lean, firm, and meaty fish. It is a fantastic source of high-quality protein with a good contribution of Omega-3s.
3. Rohu (Indian Carp)
   - Protein Content: High (approx. 16–20g per 100g).

- Omega-3 Content: Moderate (approx. 400–1000 mg per 100g).
- Ranking: A healthy, affordable source of high-quality protein, though its Omega-3 content is lower than the saltwater varieties (Rawas and Surmai)

Learning

Fish's comprehensive nutritional profile which includes, omega-3 fatty acids, high-quality protein, and essential micronutrients—firmly establishes it as a superfood. It supports heart health, brain and nerve function, and stronger immunity. No wonder it is often called the Champion of Nutrition.

Chapter 39

Almonds, Pistachios, Walnuts - The 5-star Superfoods

The "superfood" status of nuts like Almonds, Pistachios, Walnuts, and Hazelnuts comes from a powerful combination of several key healthy nutrients which they contain.

Main nutrient groups that make nuts a powerhouse are:

1. Healthy Fats

The high content of healthy fats is arguably the most defining feature. These fats, including Oleic Acid (common in almonds and hazelnuts), help lower LDL cholesterol and reduce the risk of heart disease. Walnuts are the most significant source of plant-based Omega-3 ALA, which is crucial for brain health and reducing chronic inflammation.

2. Fiber

Nuts are a great source of both soluble and insoluble fibre. Fiber supports a healthy digestive system, promotes a feeling of satiety, which aids in weight management, and helps to regulate blood sugar levels.

3.Protein

Nuts provide a significantly high amount of protein compared to other plant-based foods. Protein is essential for muscle repair, energy, and overall cell function. Almonds and Pistachios are particularly good sources of protein.

4. Essential Vitamins & Minerals

Nuts are rich in several crucial micronutrients as indicated in the following table:

Nutrient	Primary Benefit	Top Nut(s)
Vitamin E	A powerful antioxidant that protects cells from damage and supports skin and eye health.	Almonds (highest) and Hazelnuts
Magnesium	Involved in hundreds of body processes, including muscle and nerve function, blood sugar control, and blood pressure regulation.	Almonds, Cashews, Walnuts
Potassium	An electrolyte that helps manage blood pressure and is essential for heart function.	Pistachios
B Vitamins	Group of vitamins (like Folate and B6) essential for energy production and brain function.	Pistachios

5. Antioxidants and Phytochemicals

Nuts contain various beneficial plant compounds, Polyphenols, which combat oxidative stress and chronic inflammation. Pistachios are famous for their unique antioxidants like lutein and zeaxanthin, which are great for eye health. In essence, these key nutrients work together to support heart health, brain function, and metabolic health.

Nutritional Content of Nuts (per 50g)

Item	Calories	Total Fat	Saturated Fat	Unsaturated Fat	Protein	Fiber	Carbs
Almonds	289 kcal	25g	2g	23g	11g	6g	10g
Walnuts	327 kcal	33g	3g	30g	8g	3g	7g
Pistachios	281–310 kcal	23–24g	3g	20–21g	10–11g	5g	15g

Item	Calories	Total Fat	Saturated Fat	Unsaturated Fat	Protein	Fiber	Carbs
Avocados	80–122 kcal	7–12g	1–2.4g	6–9.6g	1g	3g	4g
Peanuts	283–298 kcal	24–25g	3–4g	20–22g	13–15g	4–5g	8g
Hazelnuts	176 kcal	17g	1.5g	15g	4.2g	3g	8g

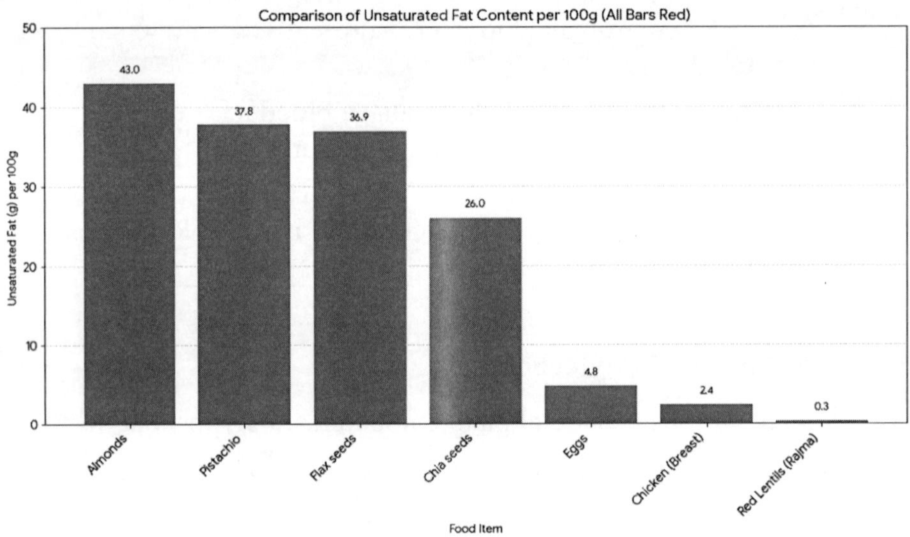

Nuts support both sleep quality and muscle rebuilding during the night.

A small handful of nuts (like walnuts, almonds, or pistachios) consumed an hour or two before bed works as a dual-action snack: the Melatonin and Magnesium help quiet the mind and induce sleep, while the Protein and Healthy Fats provide the building blocks and sustained energy for muscle repair throughout the night. Melatonin is the hormone that regulates your sleep-wake cycle (circadian rhythm). Pistachios and Walnuts are particularly high in naturally occurring melatonin. Almonds are excellent sources of magnesium. Magnesium helps to calm the nervous system and promotes muscle relaxation, linked to better sleep quality. It can help alleviate feelings of restlessness that disrupt sleep. Nuts Aid Muscle Rebuilding During Sleep. While you sleep, your body enters its most critical phase for repair and growth, a process known as muscle protein synthesis. Nuts provide a sustained release of protein. When combined with other components of an evening snack (like yogurt or whole grains), they ensure your body has the materials it needs throughout the night to perform muscle protein synthesis. The monounsaturated and polyunsaturated fats in all nuts, especially the Omega-3 ALA in Walnuts, provide the sustained energy that fuels the cellular repair processes happening in the background.

Guidelines for consuming Nuts

Since nuts have high-calorie density, one has to be careful and avoid over eating. It is better to stick to a daily serving of one ounce (28 grams). Always select raw, roasted, unsalted nuts. Avoid salted or flavoured nuts.

For nuts like Almonds and Walnuts, soaking them in water overnight and then draining helps reduce phytic acid, which can inhibit the absorption of minerals like zinc and iron, making them easier to digest.

Since each nut offers a slightly different nutrient profile, mixing of nuts ensures a broader spectrum of vitamins, minerals, and fatty acids.

While a few nuts can be a great addition to a light bedtime snack for better sleep, consume the majority of your daily portion during the morning or mid-day. Their protein and fibre combination provides sustained energy and satiety throughout the day.

Super healthy evening Snack to support Sleep and Muscle rebuilding during the night.

Basic ingredients: Almonds, Pistachios, Walnuts, milk, blueberries/straw berries/ grated apple

Take 15 g of each nut and slice or rough chop. Add 100 ml milk and warm a bit. Add blueberries/strawberries/ grated apple. Add a dash of cinnamon. Best to have it an hour before bedtime.

Health benefits: Pistachios and Walnuts are rich sources of Melatonin (sleep hormone). This directly signals the body that it is time to sleep and helps regulate your sleep-wake cycle (circadian rhythm).
Almonds & Pistachios have Magnesium which helps calm the nervous system, aids in muscle relaxation, helps you to mentally "switch off." Blueberries and Strawberries are packed with antioxidants and anti-inflammatory compounds which reduce inflammation and make muscle repair to happen more effectively. The nuts and milk provide a complete profile of essential amino acids, which are the building blocks required to repair and build muscles.

This snack provides the essential chemical signals to fall asleep easily while simultaneously delivering the building blocks for your body to repair and build muscles during sleep.

Chapter 40

Chia seeds, Flax seeds, Pumpkin seeds-The Hidden Gems

Seeds like Chia, Flax, Pumpkin, and Sesame seeds contain astonishing concentration of specific, hard-to-find micronutrients and powerful compounds, packed into such tiny, overlooked small grains.
Seeds offer a potent combination of Healthy Fats, Fiber, and unique Micronutrients that deliver major health benefits. The most potent nutrients they contain are as follows:

1-Plant-Based Omega-3 Fatty Acids (ALA)

This is the crowning feature of Chia and Flax seeds. Benefit: ALA is crucial for heart health, reducing inflammation, and is the precursor for the body to make small amounts of EPA and DHA (the Omega-3s found in fish). To absorb the ALA in Flax seeds, they must be ground before consumption, as the whole seed shell is indigestible. Chia seeds, however, can be eaten whole.

2-Exceptional Fiber Content

Seeds are one of the most fibre-dense foods available.
Soluble Fiber (high in chia and flax) forms a gel in the stomach, which slows digestion, aids blood sugar regulation, promotes satiety (feeling full), and helps lower LDL ("bad") cholesterol.
Insoluble Fiber promotes digestive regularity and bowel health.

3-Unique Minerals (Zinc & Magnesium)

Different seeds are excellent sources of minerals that are often deficient in modern diets.

Magnesium (High in Pumpkin and Chia): Essential for over 300 body processes, including nerve and muscle function, blood pressure regulation, and bone health. Its role in muscle relaxation also supports better sleep.

Zinc (High in Pumpkin Seeds): Vital for immune system support, wound healing, and is especially important for male reproductive health.

Calcium (High in Sesame Seeds): Crucial for bone density and muscle contraction. Sesame seeds, particularly unhulled ones, are one of the best non-dairy sources.

4-Specialized Antioxidants (Lignans & Sesamin)

These compounds offer targeted, powerful protection.

Lignans (High in Flax and Sesame Seeds): These are polyphenols that act as strong antioxidants. Lignans are studied for their potential to help balance hormone levels (due to a mild estrogen-mimicking effect, beneficial for menopausal women) and combat oxidative stress.

Phytosterols (High in Pumpkin Seeds): Plant compounds that have a chemical structure similar to cholesterol, allowing them to compete with and block cholesterol absorption in the gut, which helps lower blood cholesterol.

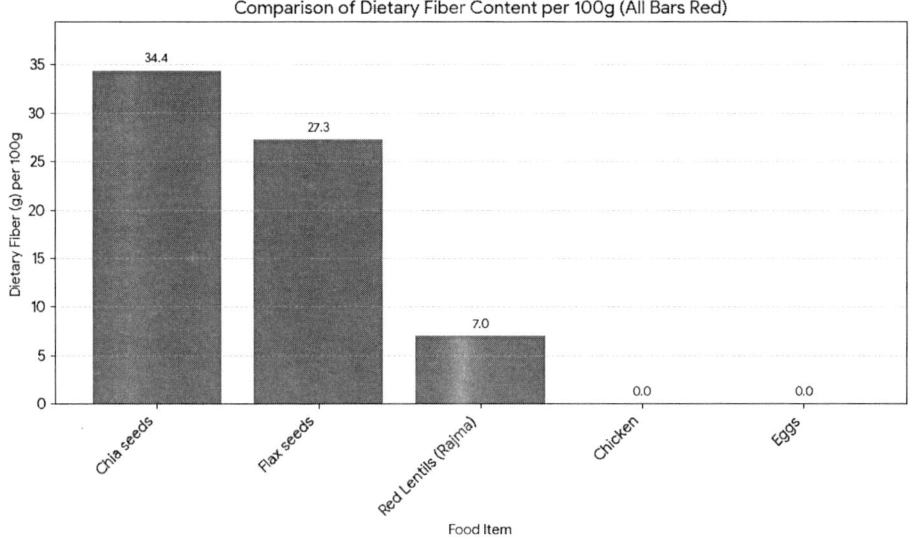

Speciality of different seeds:

Seed	Top Nutrient	Unique Health Benefit
Chia Seeds	Omega-3 ALA, Soluble Fiber, Calcium	Absorbs up to 10x its weight in water, promoting hydration and sustained energy.
Flax Seeds	Lignans, Omega-3 ALA, Soluble Fiber	Unmatched source of Lignans, beneficial for hormonal balance and cholesterol reduction. Must be ground for absorption.
Pumpkin Seeds	Zinc, Magnesium, Tryptophan	Excellent for immune function and supporting prostate health (due to zinc).
Sesame Seeds	Calcium, Lignans (	Key role in bone health (with shell) , often consumed as tahini.

These small packages are truly hidden gems because you only need a small quantity (typically 1–2 tablespoons per day) to deliver a massive health boost to your diet.

How to add popular seeds to different meals easily:

Breakfast

Seed	Preparation & Tips	Daily Meal Application
Chia Seeds	Soak in liquid to form a gel, or use dry.	Overnight Oats/Pudding: Mix 2-3 tablespoons with milk/yogurt and let sit overnight. Smoothies: Blend 1-2 teaspoons directly into your morning smoothie.
Ground Flaxseeds	Must be ground to be digestible; whole seeds pass through undigested.	Oatmeal & Cereal: Stir 1 tablespoon into your hot oatmeal or sprinkle over cold cereal/granola. Pancakes/Waffles: Add 1-2 tablespoons to the batter.
Hemp Seeds (Hemp Hearts)	Use straight out of the package—no grinding or soaking needed.	Yogurt/Cottage Cheese: Sprinkle 1 tablespoon on top for a nutty crunch and protein boost. Toast: Sprinkle over avocado or nut butter toast.
Pumpkin Seeds (Pepitas)	Toast them lightly for enhanced flavor.	Granola: Add a handful to your homemade or store-bought granola mix.
Sunflower Seeds	Toast for flavor.	Scrambled Eggs: Toss a few into your egg scramble or omelet before cooking.

For Lunch & Dinner

Seed	Preparation & Tips	Daily Meal Application
Hemp, Pumpkin, Sunflower	Raw or lightly toasted.	Salads: Sprinkle on top of any salad for texture and nutrients.
Ground Flaxseeds	Use as a binding agent or thickener.	Meatballs & Meatloaf: Use as a binder instead of breadcrumbs (1 tbsp ground flax + 3 tbsp water = 1 egg). Soups & Stews: Whisk a teaspoon into thick soups or stews right before serving.
Chia Seeds	Use ground or whole.	Dressings & Sauces: Add a pinch to salad dressings, sauces, or vinaigrettes to help them thicken slightly.
Sesame Seeds	White or black; often toasted.	Stir-fries: Sprinkle over finished stir-fries, especially Asian-inspired dishes. Steamed Veggies: Toss with steamed green beans or broccoli along with a little soy sauce or olive oil.

Snacks and Baking

Seed	Preparation & Tips	Daily Meal Application
Chia & Flaxseeds	Use as an egg substitute in baking.	Baking: Mix 1 tbsp of ground seed with 3 tbsp of water, let it sit for a few minutes until gelled, and use it in place of one egg in muffins, cookies, or quick breads.
Pumpkin & Sunflower Seeds	Use as a topping or mix-in.	Trail Mix: Mix with nuts and dried fruit. Muffins/Breads: Fold into batter or press into the top before baking.
Hemp Seeds	Can be mixed with spices.	Energy Balls/Bars: Combine with dates, oats, and nut butter to roll into no-bake energy bites.
Poppy Seeds	Often used for decoration and	Baked Goods Topping: Sprinkle on bagels, rolls, or lemon loaves before

Seed	Preparation & Tips	Daily Meal Application
	flavour.	baking.

General Tips for consuming seeds:

It is important to start eating seeds with a small quantity. Just add 1or 2 teaspoons of one type of seed per day and gradually increase the amount. This is important as seeds (especially flax and chia) are very high in fibre and can cause digestive upset if you consume too much too fast.

Always increase your water intake when adding more fibre-rich seeds to your diet and make sure that you are always hydrated.

Seeds should be stored (especially flax and chia) in the refrigerator or freezer to prevent the healthy oils from turning rancid.

Nutritional Content of Seeds (per 50g)

Seed Type	Calories	Total Fat	Saturated Fat	Unsaturated Fat	Protein	Fiber
Flax Seeds	267 kcal	21g	2g	19g	9g	14g
Chia Seeds	243 kcal	15g	2g	13g	8g	17g
Sesame Seeds	287 kcal	25g	3g	22g	9g	6g
Pumpkin Seeds	275 kcal	23g	3g	19g	14g	6g
Soy (Granules/Chunks)	345 kcal	0.5g	0g	0.5g	52g	13g

An Amazing Way to Consume Chia Seeds, Flax Seeds and Pumpkin Seeds in One shot

Basic Ingredients: 40 gm Rolled Oats+ 1 table spoon Pumpkin seeds+ 1 table spoon Chia seeds+ 1 tablespoon of ground Flax seeds.

Mix the ingredients. Add 500 ml water. Heat to boil and simmer for 10 minutes. Add 100 ml milk, half teaspoon of Cinnamon powder, one tablespoons of honey and few resins. Your delicious porridge is ready.

It provides Polyunsaturated Fats and Monounsaturated Fats including Omega-3. Cinnamon, Raisins, Honey provide Antioxidants (Polyphenols). Seeds (Pumpkin, Chia, Flax) provide Vitamin K, Vitamin E, Magnesium, Zinc, Iron, Phosphorus, and Manganese. Oats provide Vit B12, Iron and Magnesium.

This porridge is far more than just a convenient breakfast; it is a nutritionally complete meal promoting sustained energy, heart health, and robust cellular function.

Chapter 41

Prebiotic & Probiotic Foods for Gut health

Prebiotics and probiotics work hand-in-hand to promote gut health, digestion and bowel health. Our gut microbiome is a vast community of trillions of microorganisms including bacteria, viruses, fungi, and other microbes, mainly living in large intestine.

A healthy and balanced gut microbiome plays a crucial role:
-*Digesting Food*: Helps break down complex carbohydrates, fibres, and proteins that our body alone cannot digest.
-*Producing Vital Nutrients*: Some gut bacteria produce vitamins like B12 and K, and short-chain fatty acids that support gut health.
-*Boosting Immunity*: It regulates immune responses and guards against harmful pathogens.

What Are Probiotic Foods?

Probiotics are live, beneficial bacteria that support a healthy gut when consumed. These microbes help replenish and maintain the population of good bacteria in your digestive system.

Common Probiotic Foods

-Yogurt: Contains strains like Lactobacillus and Bifidobacterium.
-Kimchi: A spicy fermented Korean dish rich in probiotics.
-Kefir, Miso, Sauerkraut, Kombucha: All contain various strains of healthy bacteria and yeasts.

Traditional Indian Probiotic Foods

India has a rich tradition of fermented foods, many of which are natural probiotics:

- Kanji: A North Indian fermented drink made from black or red carrots, mustard seeds, and spices.
- Khatta Dhokla: A fermented rice and lentil dish from Gujarat.
- Dahi (Curd): Homemade curd is teeming with beneficial bacteria.
- Buttermilk (Chhaas/Mattha): A probiotic-rich fermented dairy drink.
- Idli & Dosa: South Indian staples made from fermented rice and lentils.
- Pickles: Traditional pickles like mango, lime, and mixed vegetables are fermented using salt and spices.
- Gundruk: Fermented leafy greens popular in Nepal and Northeastern India.
- Hawaijar: A fermented soybean delicacy from Manipur.
- Khorisa: Fermented bamboo shoots from Assam.

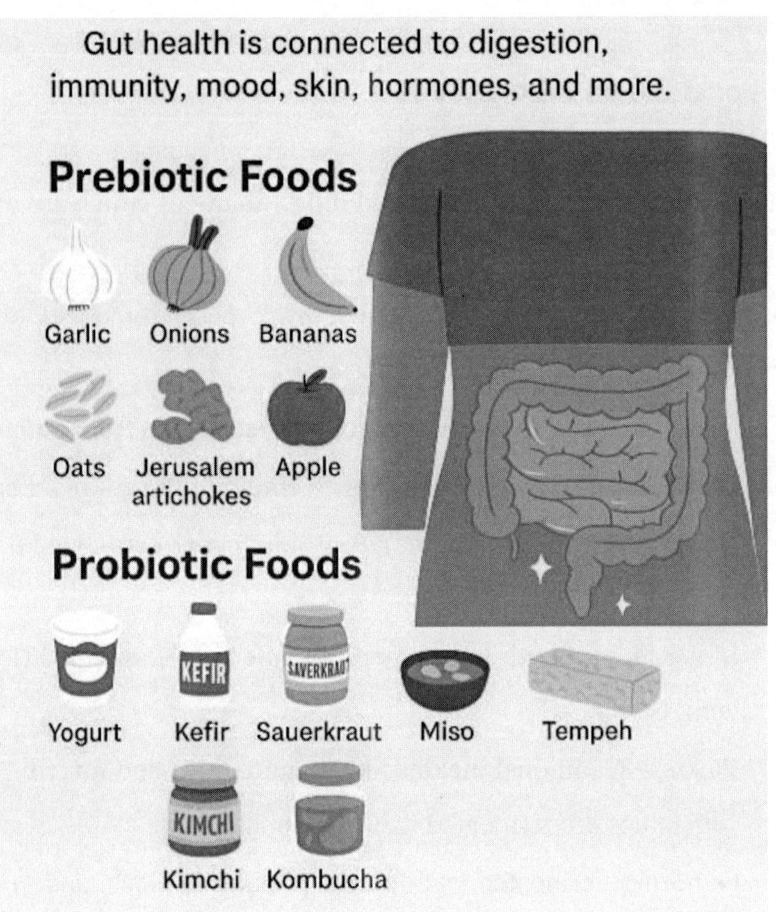

What Are Prebiotic Foods?

Prebiotics are soluble and insoluble fibres in our diet that nourish the beneficial bacteria already living in your gut. We can think of them as "food" for bacteria. They are essentially "fertilizer" that helps the "good" gut bacteria grow and thrive.

Prebiotics pass through the small intestine undigested and are then fermented by the microbes in the large intestine. This fermentation process produces beneficial compounds, like short-chain fatty acids, which support gut health and overall well-being.

A diet rich in prebiotics can help:

- Improve digestive health and regulate bowel movements.
- Enhance the growth and activity of beneficial gut flora.
- Aid in the absorption of minerals like calcium.
- Support the immune system and reduce inflammation.

Examples of Common prebiotics foods:

Garlic, onions, leeks, asparagus, bananas, oats, apples, chicory root, flaxseeds, oats, barley, Flax seeds, apples, bananas and certain legumes like beans and peas.

Learning

Prebiotic and Probiotic foods work to support a healthy gut microbiome, which is vital for overall wellness. Probiotics are live, beneficial bacteria and yeasts (found in foods like curd/yogurt, kefir, and fermented vegetables) that directly enhance the population of good microbes, aiding in digestion, improving the absorption of nutrients. Prebiotics are non-digestible fibres (found in foods like bananas, garlic, and oats) that act as food for these probiotics, selectively stimulating the growth and activity of beneficial gut bacteria. The combined consumption of both leads to an improvement in immune function (as a large portion of the immune system resides in the gut), a reduction in inflammation, and potential benefits for mood and cognitive health via the gut-brain axis.

Chapter 42

Body Weight Management – Nutritional Aspects

Managing body weight effectively is one of the most important components of maintaining good health and overall well-being. Here, we will understand the fundamentals of weight loss, the role of diet and exercise, and how to set realistic, sustainable goals.

What is Body Mass Index (BMI)?

Body Mass Index (BMI) is a numerical value derived from an individual's weight and height. It is commonly used to assess whether a person has a healthy body weight relative to their height.

How to Calculate Your BMI

Formula: BMI = Weight (kg) / (Height in meters) ^{2}

Example: If you weigh 60 kg and your height is 5 feet 4 inches (1.62 meters), BMI = 60 / (1.62 × 1.62) = 22.8 (approximately 23)

BMI Interpretation

-Less than 18.5: Underweight

-18.5 to 24.9: Healthy weight

-25 to 29.9: Overweight

-30 or above: Obese

Being overweight results in excess body fat, which increases the risk of serious health conditions such as cardiovascular diseases, type- 2 diabetes etc.

Why Exercise alone cannot result in Weight Loss

It is a common misconception that regular workouts alone are sufficient for shedding excess weight. However, both scientific evidence and real-world experience show that exercise must be paired with a reduction in calorie intake to be truly effective.

While physical activity does burn calories and improves metabolism, the number of calories burned is often less than expected. For instance, an hour of brisk walking may burn only 250–300 calories—roughly equivalent to a small snack. If calorie intake remains high, the body stores the excess energy as fat, regardless of exercise.

On the other hand, reducing daily calorie intake creates a direct energy deficit. When the body receives fewer calories than it needs, it begins to burn stored fat for fuel, leading to weight loss. In fact, approximately 80% of weight loss comes from dietary changes, while only 20% is attributed to exercise.

How to Achieve Weight Loss

Weight loss occurs when you consistently consume fewer calories than you burn—this is known as a calorie deficit. A safe and sustainable target is 0.5 to 1 kg per week, which helps prevent muscle loss and reduces stress on internal organs. To achieve this, aim for a daily calorie deficit of around 500 calories.

Effective Weight Loss Strategies

-Consume fewer calories than you expend.

-Eat a balanced diet rich in: Lean proteins, Healthy fats, High-fiber foods, Fresh vegetables and fruits

-Avoid processed, packaged, and junk foods

-Engage in at least 60 minutes of daily physical activity, including Strength training, Aerobic exercises (Zone 2 cardio), Yoga and Pranayama.

The 5-2-1-0 Rule for Weight loss

The 5-2-1-0 Rule was primarily developed for obesity prevention in children and adolescents and is widely promoted by paediatric and public health organizations.

However, the core components of the 5-2-1-0 rule are based on universal healthy lifestyle principles, which make them highly applicable and beneficial for adults undergoing a weight loss program.

The 5-2-1-0 rule translates into simple, actionable habits that directly support the calorie deficit and overall wellness required for successful adult weight loss.

- Eat 5 or More Servings of Fruits & Vegetables Daily
- Limit Screen Time to 2 Hours or Less of Recreational Use Daily
- Get 1 Hour or More of Physical Activity Daily
- Drink 0 Sugar-Sweetened Beverages

Dietary Restrictions for Weight Loss

A successful weight loss program focuses on reducing overall calorie intake while maximizing nutrient density. This often involves reducing or eliminating foods that are high in calories, unhealthy fats, and added sugars, and low in essential nutrients like fibre and protein.

Foods to Totally avoid (or minimize as much as possible)

These foods generally offer very little nutritional value while being extremely high in calories, unhealthy fats, and added sugars, making them the biggest hurdlers of a weight loss effort.

1. Sweets and Sugary Drinks such as *Soda, packaged fruit juices, energy drinks*.

Reasons to avoid: Empty Calories & Liquid Sugar. They are calorie-dense but provide no satiety (fullness), leading to massive overconsumption of sugar and calories. They are strongly linked to weight gain and metabolic disease.

2. Deep-Fried Foods such as *French fries, chips, fried chicken, donuts, and many fast-food items.*

Reasons to avoid: Trans & Unhealthy Fats. They are soaked in oil, drastically increasing calorie content and often containing unhealthy trans or saturated fats that promote inflammation and heart risk.

3. Ultra-Processed Snacks such as *packaged cookies, cakes, pastries, candy, crisps, many mass-produced granola bars.*

Reasons to avoid: Refined Carbs, Sugar, & Additives. They are designed to be hyper-palatable (easy to overeat) and are high in refined flour, added sugars, and unhealthy fats.

4. Processed Meats such as *Bacon, sausage, hot dogs, deli meats (salami, bologna).*

Reasons to avoid: High Sodium & Saturated Fat. They are high in calories, unhealthy fats, and often contain nitrates and excessive sodium, which can hinder heart and overall health.

Foods to Restrict

These foods are not necessarily "bad" but are very calorie-dense or contain refined carbohydrates that can spike blood sugar, making it harder to manage hunger and maintain a calorie deficit. Focus on smaller portions and nutrient-dense alternatives.

Food Category	**Foods to be restricted**	**Preferred alternative**
Refined Grains	White bread, white pasta, white rice, breakfast cereals with added sugar.	Whole Grains: Whole-wheat bread/pasta, brown rice, quinoa, oats. They contain fiber to keep you full longer.
High-Calorie Condiments/Sauces	Creamy salad dressings (Ranch, Thousand Island), mayonnaise, excessive butter/ghee, high-sugar ketchup.	Low-Calorie Alternatives: Vinegar, mustard, hot sauce, lemon juice, salsa, hummus, small amounts of olive oil.
Full-Fat Dairy	Whole milk, rich/creamy cheese,	Low-Fat/No-Sugar Alternatives: Skim milk,

Food Category	Foods to be restricted	Preferred alternative
	high-fat yogurt (with added sugar).	Greek yogurt (plain), cottage cheese, reduced-fat cheese in moderation.
Dried Fruit	Raisins, cranberries, dates (especially those with added sugar).	Fresh/Frozen Fruit: Berries, apples, oranges. Dried fruit is very high in concentrated sugar and calories due to the lack of water.
Alcohol	Beer, sugary cocktails, wine (especially in large quantities).	Limit Intake: Alcohol adds empty calories and can lower inhibitions, leading to poor food choices. Stick to very small, infrequent amounts or avoid completely.

Indian Foods which are forbidden

1. Indian Sweets (Mithai): Gulab Jamun, Jalebi, Laddoo, Halwa, Barfi, Peda, Rasgulla, Ras Malai.
2. Deep Fried Snacks: Samosa, Kachori, Vada , Bhajiyas ,Poori, Bhatura, All varieties of Namkeen.
3. Rich curries and gravies: Butter Chicken, Paneer Butter Masala, Shahi Paneer, Malai Kofta, Dal Makhani, Curries with large amounts of coconut milk, cream, cashew paste, or ghee.
4. Other popular foods: Butter Naan, Parathas, Biryani, Pulao, Sweet Lassi, Packaged Fruit Juices.

How to Lose Weight without Losing Muscle Mass

Losing weight while preserving muscle mass is achievable with the right approach:

1. Create a Moderate Calorie Deficit

Aim for a deficit of 300–500 calories per day. Avoid drastic reductions to prevent muscle loss. Target a weight loss of up to 1 kg per week

2. Prioritize Protein Intake

Consume 1 to 1.5 grams of protein per kilogram of body weight daily. Distribute protein intake evenly across meals and snacks (20–30 grams per serving). Good sources include Lean meats (chicken, turkey, beef), Eggs, Fish (salmon, tuna, cod), Dairy (yogurt, cottage cheese), Legumes (beans, lentils), Whey Protein powders etc.

Following picture shows recommended Foods with Healthy Fats including Omega3 (weight loss programme)

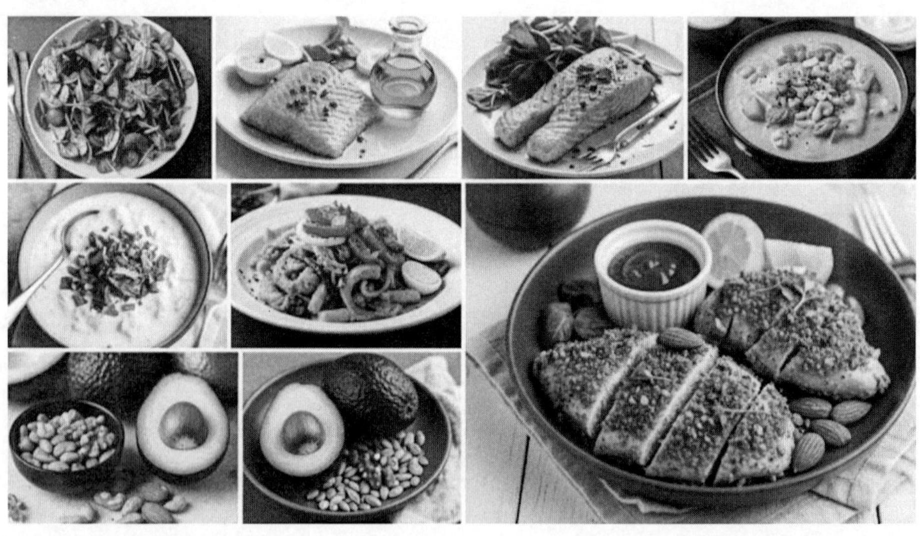

Following picture shows recommended Foods with High Protein (Weight loss programme)

Grilled Chicken Salad with avocado
High protein and fats that are good for your heart.

Quinoa Bowl with Roasted Veggies & Hummus
Plant-based, fiber-rich, and satistying

Lentil Soup
Plant-based, fiber-rich, and satisfying

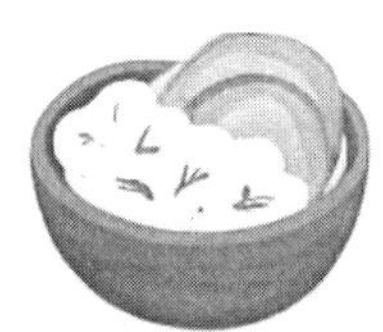

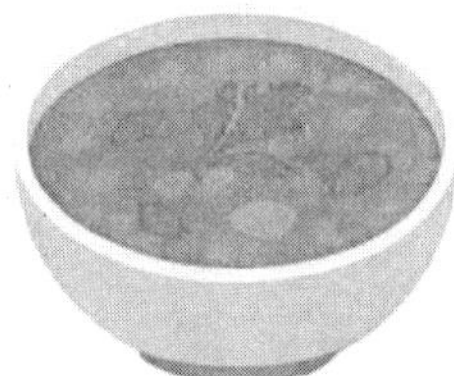

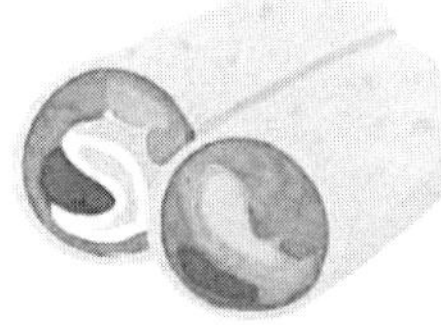

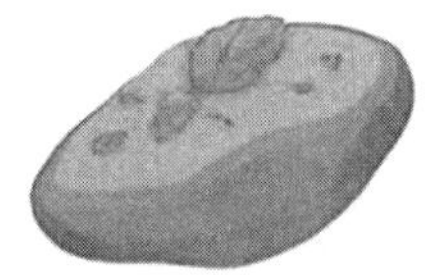

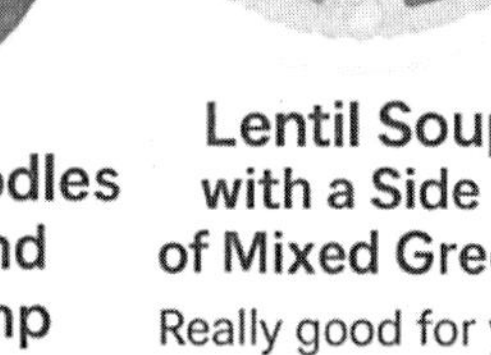

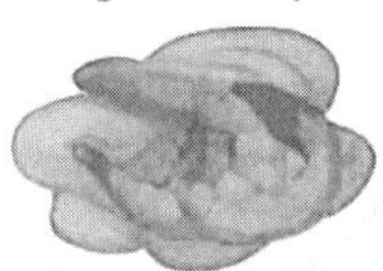

Egg Salad Lettuce Boats
High-protein and keto friendly
Chickpea Salad with Olive Oil and Lemon
Mediterranean-style, great for digestion

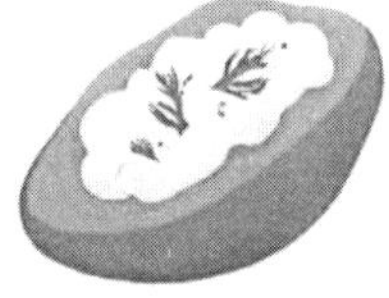

3. Include Fiber-Rich Carbohydrates

Fruits, vegetables, legumes, whole grains, nuts, seeds

4. Include Healthy Fats

Avocados, olive oil, fatty fish, nut butters

5. Do Resistance Training

Weightlifting, bodyweight exercises, resistance bands

Focus on compound movements (squats, deadlifts, bench presses)

Aim for 2–4 sessions per week

6. Do Moderate Cardiovascular Exercise

Brisk walking, cycling—150 minutes per week

High-Intensity Interval Training (HIIT) can be effective but should be done in moderation

By combining these strategies, you can effectively lose fat while maintaining lean muscle mass.

Learning:

The fundamental concept for weight loss is achieving a caloric deficit, meaning consuming fewer calories than the body expends daily. This forces the body to burn stored fat for energy. To support this deficit, the diet should prioritize nutrient-dense, whole foods—specifically high-fiber foods like vegetables, fruits, and whole grains, which promote satiety (fullness). Adequate protein intake is also crucial, as it helps preserve lean muscle mass during the calorie restriction. Conversely, success requires reducing or eliminating foods high in added sugars, unhealthy fats, and refined carbohydrates, which often contribute excess "empty" calories and hinder the deficit goal.

There is no magic bullet for weight loss. The key lies in consistently consuming fewer calories than you burn. While physical activity enhances overall health, meaningful weight loss is primarily driven by dietary changes.

Section 3

Exercises & Workouts for Longevity

Chapter 43
The Power of Physical Exercise

Physical exercise is the most potent drug for achieving a long and healthy life span. There is a positive impact of vigorous exercise virtually on every cell and organ in the body.

Why Physical Exercise is a Lifelong Necessity?

Physical exercise is not merely a choice; it is a non-negotiable pillar of lifelong health and well-being. It acts as a natural medicine for our body, mind, and spirit. The most important benefits of exercise are as follows:

Cardiovascular Health: It strengthens the heart muscle, making it more efficient at pumping blood. This lowers blood pressure, improves cholesterol profile and significantly reduces the risk of heart disease and stroke.

Metabolic Health: Exercise improves insulin sensitivity, helping to regulate blood sugar and preventing the onset of Type 2 diabetes.

Cognitive and Mental Health: Physical activity increases blood flow to the brain, which supports cognitive function, memory, and learning. It is a powerful tool for reducing symptoms of anxiety and depression by releasing mood-boosting endorphins and reducing stress hormones.

Musculoskeletal Strength: Weight-bearing exercise builds and maintains bone density, preventing osteoporosis, while strength training preserves muscle mass, which is vital for mobility and injury prevention as we age.

Why exercise becomes even more important as we age?

- As we grow older, natural physiological changes make exercise even more crucial:
- Sluggish removal of free radicals leads to cellular damage.
- Arterial hardening elevates blood pressure.
- Lung capacity declines, reducing oxygen supply to cells.
- Insulin resistance becomes common.
- Digestive issues such as constipation and piles may emerge.
- Kidney shrinkage, prostate enlargement, and a sluggish nervous system become frequent.
- Loss of muscle mass and joint degeneration often results in back pain and limited mobility.

No pill can fully prevent this biological decline. But a combination of consistent physical activity and balanced nutrition can slow it down significantly and improve quality of life.

Regular, vigorous exercise is one of the most powerful tools for ensuring good health and well-being. Ideally, people should aim for at least one hour of physical activity daily. In fact, retired seniors have the time to devote even longer to their physical exercise routines. It's important to incorporate different types of exercise because no single form can provide all the health benefits your body needs.

1. Cardiovascular Exercise

Cardiovascular (or cardio) exercises boost heart and lung function, burn calories, and improve stamina. Examples include brisk walking, jogging or running, cycling, and using a treadmill or elliptical trainer.

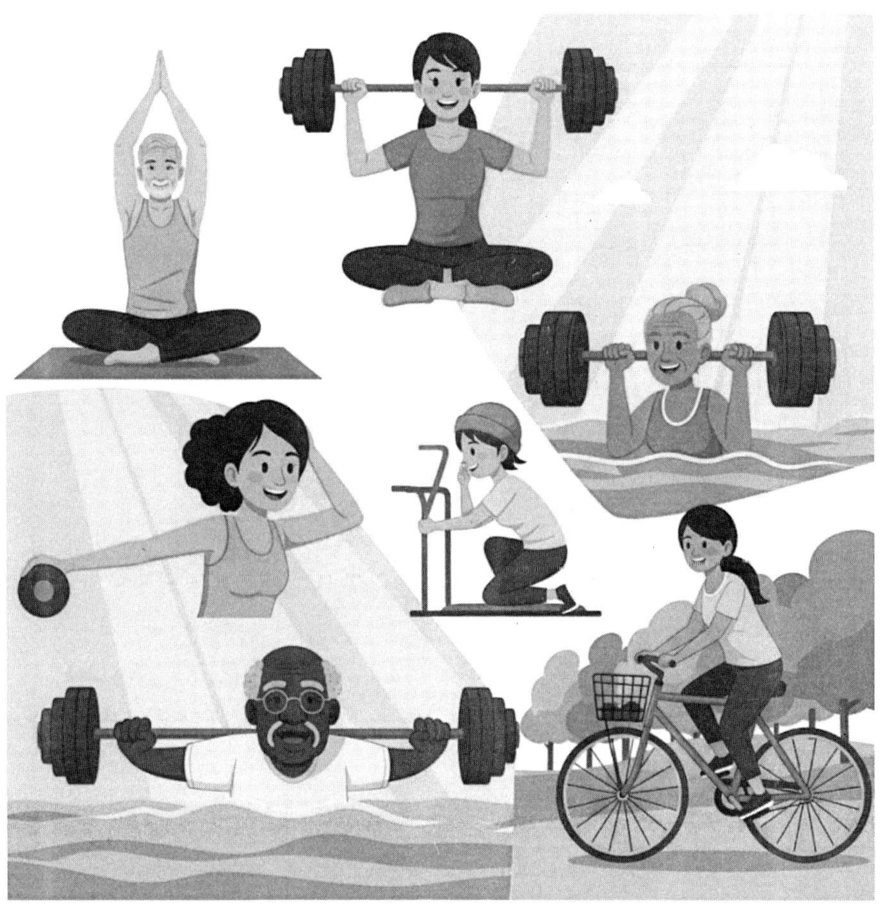

2. Strength Training

Strength training builds muscle, strengthens bones, and improves metabolism. Examples include using dumbbells, weight lifting, resistance bands, squats, lunges, push-ups, crunches, planks, and stretches like the bench press, overhead press, pull-ups, bicep curls, triceps extensions, and calf raises.

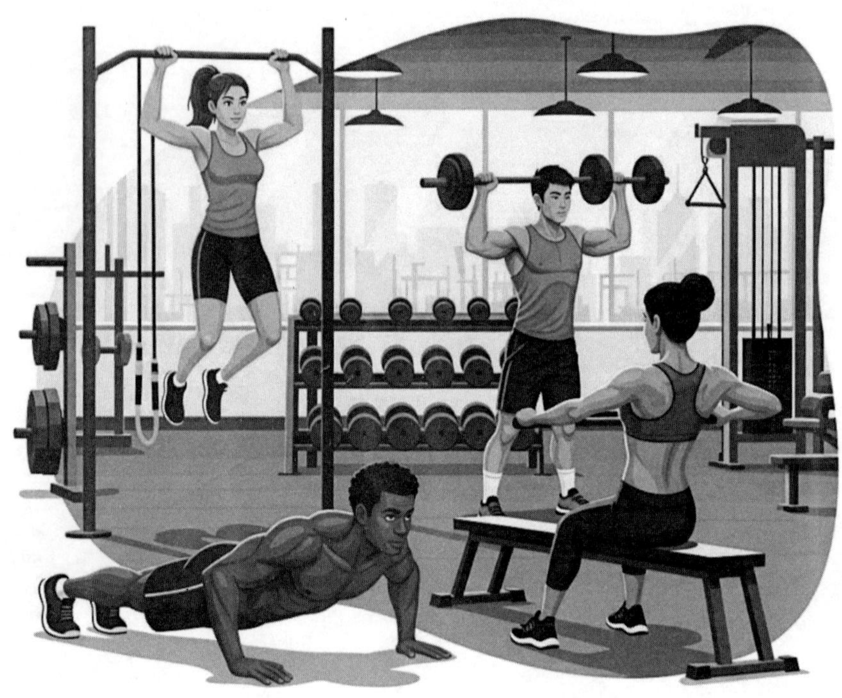

3. Flexibility and Balance Exercises

These exercises prevent stiffness, improve posture, reduce the risk of falls, and increase the range of joint movement. Examples include yoga, stretching, tai chi, Pilates, the cat-cow posture, and shoulder rolls.

A good weekly schedule combines different exercises:

Cardio: 30–40 minutes, 5–6 days per week

Strength Training: 3–4 days per week

Flexibility/Balance: Short daily sessions, such as yoga or stretching

Incorporate Resistance Training:

Resistance training (weightlifting, bodyweight exercises, and resistance bands) is the most effective way to preserve and build muscle during weight loss. Focus on compound movements that engage multiple muscle groups simultaneously, such as: Squats, Deadlifts, Bench presses, Rows, Overhead presses. Aim for 3-4 resistance training sessions per week.

Include Moderate Cardiovascular Exercise:

Cardio can help create a calorie deficit and improve overall health. Aim for moderate-intensity cardio sessions (like brisk walking or cycling) for about 150 minutes per week. High-Intensity Interval Training (HIIT) can also be effective for fat loss and may help preserve muscle, but should be used in moderation.

Learning:

Regular physical activity is scientifically proven to significantly reduce the risk of developing major chronic illnesses, including coronary heart disease, stroke, type 2 diabetes, and several cancers. It fundamentally strengthens the cardiovascular system by lowering blood pressure, improving cholesterol profiles and enhancing overall circulation. Beyond physical health, exercise offers immediate and long-term mental health benefits: it stimulates brain chemicals that improve mood, reduce feelings of anxiety and depression, sharpen cognitive skills, and significantly improve sleep quality. Furthermore, resistance training activities help maintaining bone density and muscle mass which has a significant impact on fitness and longevity.

Chapter 44

Heart Rate & Zone 2 Cardio Workouts

Zone 2 cardio workout is the most potent tool to achieve excellent cardiovascular health and extend the life expectancy.

Your heart rate is the number of times your heart beats per minute (BPM). It varies depending on factors such as age, fitness level, and physical activity. Understanding your heart rate zones can help you exercise more effectively.

What is Your Maximum Heart Rate?

This is calculated using a simple formula:

220−Your Age=Maximum Heart Rate (MHR)

For example, if you are 40 years old, your MHR is 220−40=180 bpm.

What is Your Resting Heart Rate?

This is typically between 60–100 bpm for most adults. You can measure it by placing your fingers on your wrist and counting your pulse for 60 seconds while at rest, ideally, first thing in the morning.

Understanding Heart Rate Zones

Your heart rate zones are calculated as percentages of your maximum heart rate. Each zone targets a specific intensity level and provides unique benefits:

Zone 1: Very Light (50–60% of MHR) — Ideal for warm-ups and recovery.

Zone 2: Light / Aerobic / Endurance (60–70% of MHR)

Zone 3: Moderate / Tempo (70–80% of MHR)

Zone 4: Hard / Threshold (80–90% of MHR)

Zone 5: Maximal / All-Out Effort (90–100% of MHR)

You can use your phone's calculator or a heart rate zone app to get precise values based on your age and resting heart rate.

What is Zone 2 Cardio?

Zone 2 cardio is aerobic exercise performed at 60–70% of your maximum heart rate. It's a light-to-moderate-intensity workout that improves endurance and promotes fat burning.

The Talk Test:

If you can speak comfortably in short sentences (3–5 words at a time) but can't sing, you're likely in Zone 2.

Benefits of Zone 2 Cardio

Fat Burning: At this intensity, the body uses fat as its primary energy source.

Improved Heart Health: Regular Zone 2 training enhances cardiovascular function.

Increased Endurance: It helps you sustain long-duration activities like walking, biking, or swimming.

Enhanced Oxygen Utilization: It boosts your body's ability to deliver and use oxygen efficiently.

Low Risk of Overtraining: It's gentle enough for frequent practice without causing burnout or injury.

Examples of Zone 2 Cardio Exercises

These activities should be done at a "conversational pace" where your heart rate stays within 60–70% of your MHR:

Brisk walking, Light jogging, Outdoor cycling or stationary biking, Swimming (continuous, steady-paced laps), Rowing machine, Elliptical trainer (at a steady, moderate pace)

Why Zone 2 is good for Weight Loss?

Zone 2 training is excellent for sustainable weight loss, especially when combined with a proper diet. It helps your body become more efficient at using energy and managing blood sugar. In Zone 2 (60–70% of Maximum Heart Rate), your body predominantly uses fat as its primary fuel source, which is key for long-term fat loss.

How Zone 2 Compares with Other Workouts for Weight Loss

Training Type	Fat Burn Efficiency	Calories Burned	Impact on Metabolism	Suitability
Zone 2 Cardio	High (fat burning)	Moderate	Builds aerobic base	Excellent for all levels
HIIT (High-Intensity Interval Training)	Moderate (mostly burns carbs)	High (in a short time)	Raises metabolism post-exercise (EPOC effect)	Great for time-crunched and fit individuals
Strength Training	Indirect (builds muscle, boosts BMR)	Moderate	Long-term fat loss via muscle gain	Ideal when combined with cardio

Zone 2, Cardio & HIIT for Weight Loss

The most effective and sustainable approach for weight loss combines:

Zone 2 cardio: (5times/week) to build fat-burning capacity.

Strength training: (3 times/week) to preserve and build muscle mass.

HIIT: (2 times/week) to boost calorie burn and metabolism.

If you are overweight, sedentary, or just starting, Zone 2 is the safest and most effective starting point. Once you are fitter, you can layer in other types of exercise for faster results.

Learning

Zone 2 cardio is an essential form of aerobic training that offers powerful benefits, especially for heart health, fat metabolism, and endurance. Whether you're a beginner or an experienced exerciser, incorporating Zone 2 workouts into your weekly routine can help you build a strong foundation for long-term fitness and wellness.

Chapter 45

Strength Training for Muscle Building

This is another important exercise which significantly improves cardiovascular health in addition to increasing muscle mass. Strength training, also known as resistance or weight training is a form of physical exercise in which your muscles work against an external resistance. This resistance could be weights, resistance bands, or even your own body weight. The goal is to build muscle strength, increase endurance, improve mobility, and enhance overall fitness.

Benefits of Strength Training

Strength training offers a wide range of physical, mental, and metabolic benefits that go far beyond just building muscle. Its most important advantages are as follows:

- Increases muscle strength and endurance which helps you perform daily tasks more efficiently.
- Improves bone density which reduces the risk of osteoporosis and fractures, especially in older adults.
- Enhances joint stability and flexibility which supports better posture and reduces injury risk.
- Boosts mobility and balance, especially important for aging populations to prevent falls.
- Strength training increases your resting metabolic rate, helping you burn more calories even at rest.
- Reduces abdominal fat which is linked to heart disease and diabetes.

- Improves insulin sensitivity: aids in blood sugar regulation, lowering the risk of type 2 diabetes.
- Supports cardiovascular health by improving circulation and reducing blood pressure.

Mental & Emotional Benefits of Strength Training

- It Releases endorphins which boost mood and reduce anxiety.
- Enhances self-confidence
- Improves cognitive function especially in older adults. It is linked to better memory and brain health.
- Regular training can lead to deeper, more restorative sleep.
- Slows age-related muscle loss and improves quality of life as you age.

Examples of Strength Training Workouts

Bodyweight Exercises:

Push-ups – Targets chest, shoulders, and triceps

Squats – Builds quads, glutes, and hamstrings

Planks – Strengthens core and stabilizers

Lunges – Works legs and improves balance

Pull-ups – Great for back and biceps

Free Weights (Dumbbells):

Deadlifts – Full-body strength, especially posterior chain

Bench Press – Chest, shoulders, and triceps

Overhead Press – Shoulders and upper back

Squats – Quads and glutes with core engagement

Resistance Machines:

Leg Press – Quads, hamstrings, and glutes

Chest Press – Chest and triceps

Shoulder Press Machine – Deltoids and triceps

Learning

Resistance training involves working your muscles against a force (such as weights, resistance bands, or body weight) and is crucial for increasing muscle strength and muscle mass. Further, resistance training is the most effective way to improve bone density, significantly reducing the risk of osteoporosis and fractures later in life. It also enhances balance and stability, and boosts glucose metabolism, making it a powerful tool in preventing and managing Type 2 diabetes. Overall, incorporating resistance training is essential for maintaining physical independence and improving quality of life across all ages.

Chapter 46

High-Intensity Interval Training

HIIT stands for High-Intensity Interval Training. It's an effective exercise strategy that involves alternating short bursts of very intense exercise with brief periods of rest or recovery. You can combine HIIT with Zone 2 training (low-intensity cardio) for optimal results.

How a HIIT Workout is done?

You go all-out for a short time (like sprinting or jumping jacks for 30 seconds). Then you rest or slow down (like walking or standing still for 15–30 seconds). You repeat this cycle several times, usually for about 15 to 30 minutes total.

During the high-intensity intervals, you push your body to its maximum effort. This means getting your heart rate up significantly (often 80% or more of your maximum heart rate). During this state, you would be breathless and hardly able to speak more than a few words at a time. Most aerobic exercises can fit nicely into a HIIT workout session, such as Running, Brisk walking, Cycling, Stair climbing, rowing, Calisthenics and bodyweight exercises (e.g., lunges, jumping jacks, squat jumps, and burpees).

It's generally not recommended to do HIIT workouts every day. Beginners should start with one HIIT session per week and gradually increase to 2-3 sessions. Due to its intensity, HIIT can boost your metabolism for hours after you've finished, resulting in additional calories burned even after your workout is over.

Benefits of HIIT:

- Heart Health: Research shows that getting your heart pumping more vigorously on a regular basis can help reduce high blood pressure.
- Calorie Burn: Shorter, more intense bursts of exercise can burn more calories than a slow-and-steady workout. An added perk? It takes less time, which is always a plus in a world with jam-packed schedules.
- Fat Loss: HIIT can help you lose body fat, especially if you have obesity.
- Metabolism Boost: Revving up your internal engine with HIIT has a carryover effect, as your metabolism remains elevated for hours after exercise. That helps burn calories long after you finish working out.
- Reduced Blood Sugar: Study after study shows that HIIT can reduce blood sugar and improve insulin resistance, making it an ideal option for those with Type 2 diabetes or prediabetes.

Combining HIIT Principles with Bhastrika Pranayama

Bhastrika Pranayama involves rapid and forceful inhalations and exhalations, mimicking a blacksmith's bellows. This generates heat and energy in the body, increases oxygen flow, and strengthens the respiratory system. It's often referred to as a "yogic breath of fire" due to its energizing nature.

Intensity: Bhastrika, especially at a fast pace, involves vigorous and forceful breathing, which can increase heart rate and oxygen intake, much like a high-intensity physical activity. It creates an internal "cardio-boosting" effect.

Intervals (Implicit): Traditionally, Bhastrika is practiced in rounds, with periods of forceful breathing followed by short rests or normal breathing. This naturally creates an "interval" structure.

How to Apply HIIT Principles to Bhastrika:

1. *Varying Intensity*: You could consciously vary the intensity of your Bhastrika practice. For example:

   High-intensity bursts: Perform a set number of rapid, forceful Bhastrika breaths.

   Recovery periods: Follow with a period of normal, gentle breathing or a slower, more controlled Bhastrika.

   Repeat: Cycle through these high-intensity and recovery phases.
2. *Increased Rounds/Duration*: Gradually increase the number of rounds of forceful Bhastrika or the duration of each "intense" burst, similar to how you would progress in a physical HIIT workout.
3. *Focus on "Maximal Effort" (for breathing)*: In HIIT, you push to near-maximal physical effort. With Bhastrika, this would translate to pushing your lung capacity and respiratory muscles to a high, yet safe, intensity during the active phase.

In conclusion, while Bhastrika is not a standard HIIT workout, its inherent intensity and rhythmic nature make it conducive to applying HIIT principles. By varying the intensity and duration of forceful breathing, you could potentially amplify its benefits for respiratory health, oxygenation, and overall vitality.

Learning:

While traditional resistance training builds muscle mass, the intense nature of HIIT triggers powerful hormonal responses that aid in muscle preservation and improve the body's ability to utilize energy efficiently. HIIT dramatically improves cardiovascular fitness and increases mitochondrial density (powerhouses of the cells), which slows cellular aging and improves metabolic health more effectively than steady-state cardio. This superior metabolic conditioning leads to better insulin sensitivity, reduced visceral fat, and enhanced VO2 max, all of which are key predictors of a longer, healthier life.

Chapter 47

VO2 Max & Its Importance

VO2 Max is the most significant predictor of longevity. It is the maximum amount of oxygen your body can utilize during intense exercise. A higher VO2 max means better endurance and superior cardiovascular health.

Maintaining a high VO2 max helps you stay physically independent as you age.

People with a high VO2 max are up to 5 times less likely to die from any cause compared to those with low levels.

VO2 max naturally declines with age, but you can slow or even reverse this trend through training.

A higher VO2 max is also linked to a better mood and increased happiness.

Average VO2 Max for an Active Person

The average VO2 max for an active person varies significantly with age and gender. Generally, a higher number indicates a higher level of cardiorespiratory fitness. The values below are a good reference for what is considered "Good" or "Excellent" for an active individual in each age and gender group:

Average VO2 Max for Active Men: 39 to 45

Average VO2 Max for Active Women: 30 to 40

Key Factors Influencing VO2 Max

- VO2 max naturally declines with age, even in highly active individuals.
- Men typically have a higher VO2 max than women due to physiological differences like greater muscle mass, heart size, and haemoglobin levels.
- Genetic factors can account for a significant portion of an individual's VO2 max potential.
- Since VO2 max is measured per kilogram of body weight, having a lower body fat percentage and higher lean muscle mass will generally result in a better score.

How HIIT Improves VO2 Max

HIIT is particularly effective at improving VO2 max because it pushes your body to work at a very high intensity. Here's why it's so beneficial:
It significantly boosts your body's ability to use oxygen, a key marker of cardiovascular fitness and longevity.
It provides more results in less time compared to steady-state cardio, making it ideal for time-strapped individuals.
HIIT enhances insulin sensitivity and mitochondrial function, contributing to overall metabolic health.

Learning:

VO2 max is widely considered the single best measure of cardiovascular fitness. Improving VO2 max through training, particularly HIIT, significantly enhances the efficiency of your heart, lungs, and muscles, allowing you to sustain higher intensity activities for longer. Crucially for longevity, a higher VO2 max is strongly correlated with a reduced risk of mortality and cardiovascular disease, serving as a powerful and independent predictor of long-term health. It is a powerful tool for anyone who wants to live longer, stay independent, and feel better physically and mentally.

Section 4

Human Body & Lifestyle Diseases

Chapter 48

The Immune System – How it protects you

Every day, our body is under attack from millions of bacteria, viruses, and other germs. Fortunately, we have a built-in defence force called the immune system. It works silently 24/7 to keep us safe, fighting off infections and protecting our health.

Where is it located?

Unlike the heart or lungs, the immune system is not in just one spot. It is a network spread throughout the body. It has two main parts:

1. Innate Immune System –This is the protection you are born with. It provides a quick, general defence against invaders.
2. Acquired (Adaptive) Immune System –This develops as you grow. It learns and remembers every germ it meets. The next time it encounters that same germ, it can respond faster and stronger.

This memory is the reason why you do not usually get sick from the same infection twice.

First Line of Defence:

Your body has several barriers to prevent the entry of germs.

-*Skin* – A tough outer wall.

-*Mucus in the nose and throat* – Traps microbes like sticky glue.

-*Saliva* – Washes germs away.

-*Stomach acid* – Destroys many harmful bacteria in food.

How Does the Immune System Work?

If germs slip past these barriers, special soldiers called white blood cells (lymphocytes) step in. They are circulating in your blood and lymph, always hunting for invaders. They are made in the bone marrow. They detect and destroy harmful microbes and remember past enemies. So, the next time the same germ shows up, the attack is quicker and stronger. That is the secret behind immunity.

This memory is also how vaccines work- they teach your immune system to recognise a germ without you ever getting sick from it.

How to Keep Your Immune System Strong

Think of your immune system as an army. To fight well, it needs the right care and support. You can provide it by doing the following:

- Eat plenty of fruits, vegetables, whole grains, and lean proteins. Nutrients like Vitamin C, D, zinc, and selenium are vital.
- Get enough sleep. Seven to nine hours of good sleep help your body repair and recharge.
- Manage stress – Long-term stress weakens your defence. Try exercise, meditation, nature walks, or simply spending time with loved ones.
- Stay active – Regular moderate exercise boosts circulation, helping immune cells move quickly around the body.
- Practice hygiene – Simple handwashing still works wonders!
- Get sunlight (or Vitamin D supplements) – Vitamin D is a powerful immune booster.

Consistency is the key. Small daily habits build a strong defence system.

Vitamins and Minerals for Immune Support:

Certain vitamins, minerals, and supplements play an important role in supporting and maintaining a healthy immune system.

Vitamin C: A powerful antioxidant that protects immune cells from damage; supports the production of white blood cells. May help reduce the duration and severity of the common cold, especially in high-stress individuals.

Vitamin D: Crucial for regulating the immune response; enhances the pathogen-fighting effects of immune cells. Many people are deficient, especially in low-sunlight months. Supplementation is often recommended to maintain optimal blood levels.

Vitamin A: Important for maintaining the integrity of the body's protective barriers (skin, gut lining, and respiratory tract) and for proper immune cell development. Best obtained through diet e.g., sweet potatoes, carrots, spinach.

Zinc: Known as the "gatekeeper" of the immune system. Essential for the development and activation of T-cells (key immune cells) and for wound healing. Short-term use of zinc lozenges may help shorten the duration of a cold if taken early.

Selenium: Acts as an antioxidant and is important for activating the immune system when a threat is present, while also regulating the response to prevent chronic inflammation. Found in Brazil nuts, which is a very rich source of Selenium.

Various Pro-biotics, Turmeric and Omega-3 fatty acids also support the immune health.

What triggers Autoimmune Diseases?

Sometimes, the immune system gets confused. Instead of attacking germs, it attacks the body's own healthy cells. This leads to autoimmune diseases. There can be several triggers:

- Genes (family history)
- Environmental toxins and pollution
- Certain medicines
- Lack of Vitamin D
- Gluten in celiac disease
- Chronic stress
- Smoking (a major risk factor)

Examples of Autoimmune Diseases:

- Rheumatoid Arthritis (RA): Damages joints
- Lupus: Affects skin, joints, and organs
- Psoriasis: Skin condition
- Inflammatory Bowel Disease (IBD): Affects digestion
- Multiple Sclerosis (MS): Affects nerves
- Type 1 Diabetes: Attacks insulin-producing cells
- Thyroid disorders (Graves', Hashimoto's)
- Sjögren's Syndrome: Damages tear and saliva glands

- Celiac Disease: Reaction to gluten affecting the gut

Learning:

The immune system possesses an incredible biological "memory," housed primarily in specialized memory B and T cells. Once these cells encounter a specific virus or bacteria, they keep a detailed record of its structure (antigens) for decades. This allows the immune system to launch a rapid, precise counter-attack if the same invader is encountered again. This sophisticated memory is the fundamental principle that makes vaccination possible and effective.

The immune system is one of the most remarkable systems of the body. It is always on guard, protecting you against countless threats you never see. By understanding how it works and giving it the care it deserves, you can remain healthy throughout your life.

Chapter 49

Nervous System and Homeostasis

We can think of our nervous system as the body's super-fast communication network. It allows you do everything, from running and breathing to feeling emotions and thinking deep thoughts. This amazing system keeps everything coordinated and in check, a crucial job for staying healthy.

How it functions?

It acts as a control centre and handles following key jobs:

Receiving Signals: It acts like a sensor, picking up info from your eyes, ears, and skin. For example, it's what makes you pull your hand away from a hot stove.

Processing Info: It is the brain's job to make sense of all this incoming data and decide what to do next.

Sending Instructions: It sends out commands to your muscles and glands, telling them how to react—like telling your arm muscles to move.

Keeping things stable: It is the master of homeostasis, which is the body's incredible ability to maintain a stable internal balance, like keeping your body temperature just right, no matter the weather outside.

Thinking and feeling: This is where all your memories, thoughts, and feelings come from.

Main Parts of the Nervous system

Your nervous system has a few main components that work together flawlessly:

Brain: The ultimate command centre, which processes information, makes decisions, and initiates all your actions.

Spinal Cord: A superhighway of nerves that connects your brain to the rest of your body, sending messages back and forth.

Nerves: These are the communication cables that link your brain and spinal cord to every single part of your body.

Branches of Nervous System

The whole system is split into two branches, Central Nervous System and Peripheral Nervous System. Central nervous system consists of your brain and spinal cord—the main processing hub. All the important decisions are made here. Peripheral nervous system includes all the nerves that branch out from the Central Nervous System, reaching your limbs and organs. It acts as the bridge connecting your control centre to the rest of your body.

The Peripheral Nervous System has two parts: First is *Somatic Nervous System* which can be considered as the "conscious control" system. It handles all your voluntary movements, like picking up a book or kicking a ball. The second is *Autonomic Nervous System.* It controls all the involuntary functions like beating of heart or digestion of food.

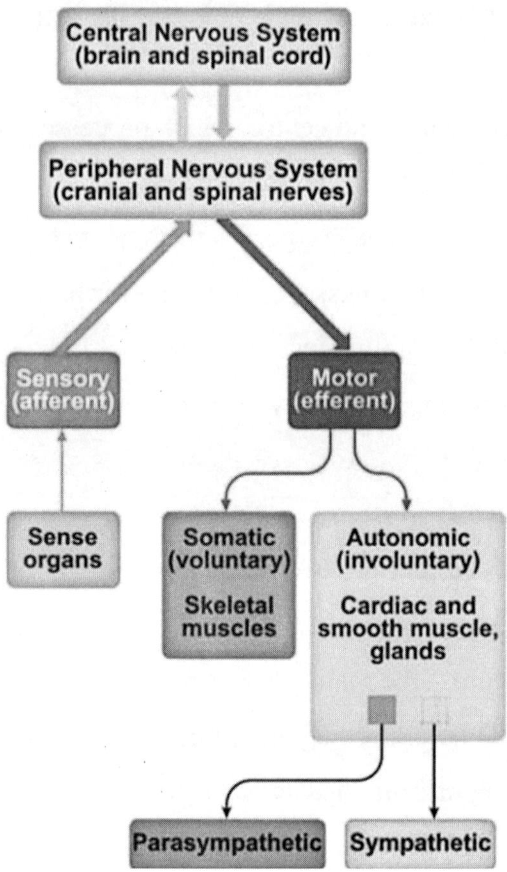

The Autonomic Nervous System

The Autonomic Nervous System has two divisions that are constantly working to keep you balanced, like a car's accelerator and brake pedal. This is the nervous system's key to maintaining homeostasis.

Sympathetic Nervous System: "Fight or Flight"

This system quickly prepares you for action. When you are in a stressful situation, it kicks in, increasing your heart rate, dilating your pupils, and pumping out adrenaline. It gets your body ready to either fight the threat or run away from it.

Parasympathetic Nervous System: "Rest and Digest"

This system puts your body in cool-down mode. After the stress is gone, it takes over to calm you down. It lowers your heart rate, promotes digestion, and helps you conserve and restore energy.

Sympathetic System (Accelerator)	**Parasympathetic System (Brake)**
Increases heart rate	Decreases heart rate
Dilates pupils	Constricts pupils
Inhibits digestion	Stimulates digestion
Releases adrenaline	Conserves energy
Mobilizes energy for action	Promotes calmness and recovery

What diseases are caused when it goes wrong?

Sometimes, this incredible system can have problems. Disorders of the nervous system can cause serious diseases like:

- Alzheimer's disease: A progressive condition that causes memory loss and confusion.
- Parkinson's disease: A disorder that affects movement, leading to tremors and stiffness.
- Multiple Sclerosis (MS): This condition damages the protective coating on your nerves, disrupting messages and causing a variety of symptoms.
- Epilepsy: Causes seizures due to abnormal electrical activity in the brain.

Learning

The Nervous System is the body's super-fast communication network. It transmits signals via electrical and chemical waves that can travel at speeds exceeding 220 miles per hour. This extraordinary speed is essential for critical functions, such as enabling you to instantly jerk your hand away from a hot surface or sending the motor commands necessary for complex muscle coordination.

Your nervous system is the ultimate command and control centre, co-ordinating everything from your simple reflexes to your most complex thoughts. It works closely to keep your body in a state of perfect harmony, adapting to every change inside and out. Understanding it is key to appreciating just how your body stays healthy and in balance.

Chapter 50

Endocrine System & Liver

The endocrine system is like your body's hormonal command centre. Endocrine glands release tiny chemical messengers called hormones directly into the blood. These hormones travel all over the body and control important functions such as growth and development, energy and metabolism, mood and emotions, stress response and reproduction

The key Endocrine glands are:

1. Hypothalamus (the coordinator and controller)
2. Pineal gland
3. Pituitary (the "master gland")
4. Thyroid
5. Parathyroid
6. Thymus
7. Adrenal glands
8. Pancreas
9. Ovaries (females)
10. Testes (males)

The *hypothalamus* is the co-ordinator and controller of endocrine system. It tells the pituitary and other glands when to switch on or off. It is also a link between the nervous system and the endocrine system.

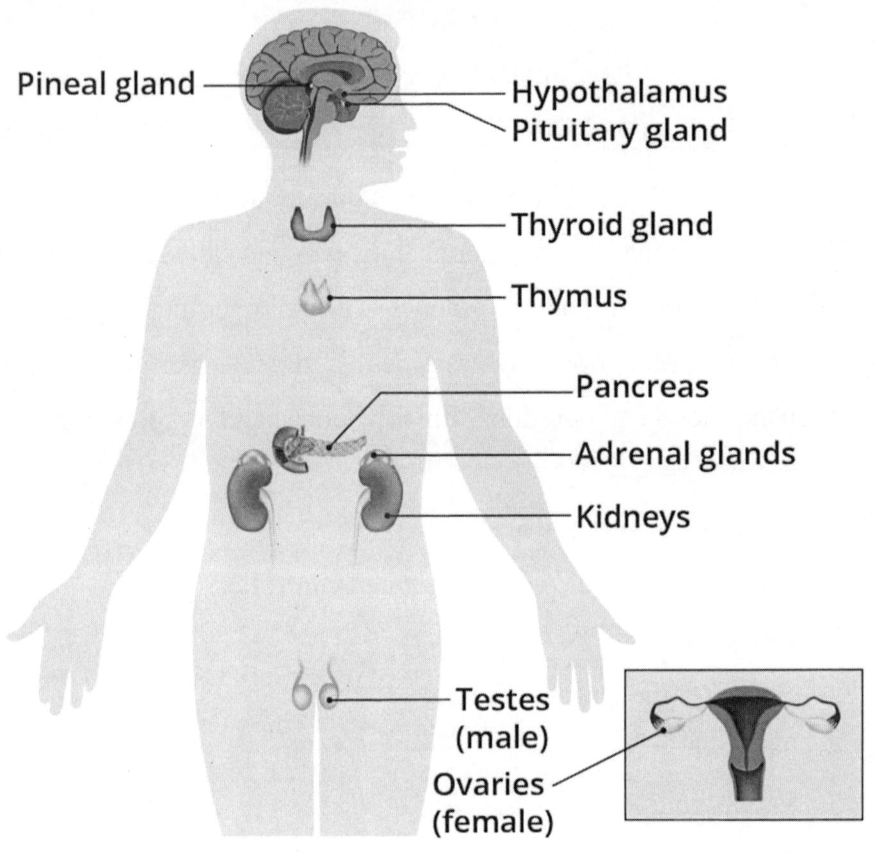

Major Hormones and their Functions

Hypothalamus releases hormones which regulate hunger, thirst, body temperature, and daily rhythms. It signals the pituitary to act. It also produces oxytocin and Dopamine.

Pituitary (Master Gland): Releases hormones that control growth, thyroid activity, reproduction, and other glands.

Thyroid: Produces T3 and T4 hormones to regulate metabolism, energy, and growth.

Adrenal Glands-

Outer layer (Cortex): Produces cortisol (stress and metabolism regulator).

Inner layer (Medulla): Produces adrenaline and noradrenaline for the "fight or flight" response.

Pancreas: Produce Insulin and Glucagon to keeps blood sugar balanced.

Insulin lowers blood sugar.

Glucagon raises blood sugar.

Ovaries (Females): Produce oestrogen for menstrual cycles and reproduction.

Testes (Males): Produce testosterone for male development and fertility.

Pineal Gland : Produces melatonin, the sleep–wake cycle hormone.

Functions of Key Organs

Pancreas

The pancreas serves a dual function of digesting food and regulating blood sugar.

The pancreas produces two important hormones Insulin and Glucagon.

Insulin (from beta cells): moves sugar into cells, lowers blood glucose, stores extra sugar as glycogen.

Glucagon (from alpha cells): releases stored sugar from the liver when levels are low.

Insulin lowers blood sugar and Glucagon raises blood sugar.

Together, insulin and glucagon keep your blood sugar steady, like a thermostat balancing room temperature.

Adrenal Glands

Adrenal glands are a pair of small triangular-shaped glands located on top of each kidney. Each gland consists of two distinct parts; the outer Cortex and the inner Medulla. The cortex produces steroid hormone Cortisol which regulates metabolism and stress response. The medulla produces adrenaline and noradrenalin which are crucial for the fight-or-flight response.

What role played by Adrenal gland in Fight or Flight response?

When you face a sudden, stressful situation—like a near car accident or a scary encounter—your body activates the 'fight or flight' response to help you react quickly. The adrenal glands play a key role in this response:

Your brain detects a threat and signals the adrenal glands.

The adrenal glands release adrenaline and noradrenaline into the bloodstream.

These hormones trigger quick changes in your body to help you either 'fight' the danger or 'flee' from it:

Heart Rate Increases – more blood and oxygen are sent to your muscles.

Breathing Speeds Up – your lungs take in more oxygen.

Energy Boosts – stored sugar (glucose) is released for a quick energy supply.

Muscles Tense and become ready to react physically.

Pupils Dilate – your vision sharpens to detect danger.

Blood is directed to essential muscles and away from non-essential functions (like digestion).

As soon as the danger is over, your adrenal glands stop releasing these hormones, and your body gradually returns to its normal state.

Liver – The Chemical Factory

Liver is not a part of Endocrine System. But it plays an extremely important role. The liver sits in the upper right side of the abdomen, just below the diaphragm. It is about the size of a football. The liver plays a crucial role in metabolism, detoxification, and nutrient processing. Hence it is called the body's 'chemical factory.'

Major functions:

1. Balances blood sugar (stores glucose as glycogen, releases it when needed)
2. Produces bile to digest fats
3. Detoxifies harmful substances like alcohol and drugs
4. Processes nutrients from food
5. Regulates cholesterol and hormones
6. Produces proteins that are important for blood clotting and fluid balance

How the Liver Balances Blood Sugar Levels?

The liver acts as the body's central glucose reservoir and factory, constantly working with the pancreatic hormones insulin and glucagon to keep blood sugar levels stable within a narrow, healthy range.

When Blood Sugar is high (After a Meal)

- The pancreas releases Insulin.

- Insulin signals the liver to absorb excess glucose from the bloodstream.
- The liver then converts this glucose into its storage form, glycogen, through a process called Glycogenesis.
- The liver essentially acts as a buffer, removing and storing the surplus sugar.

When Blood Sugar is Low (Between Meals or Fasting)

- The pancreas releases Glucagon.
- Glucagon signals the liver to release glucose back into the bloodstream.
- The liver achieves this through two main processes:
    1. Glycogenolysis: Breaking down the stored glycogen back into glucose.
    2. Gluconeogenesis: Manufacturing new glucose from non-carbohydrate sources (like amino acids and lactate).

By constantly balancing these processes of glucose storage and production, the liver ensures a steady energy supply, especially for the brain, which relies almost entirely on glucose for fuel.

In short, the liver is your body's metabolism manager plus a detox plant plus an energy warehouse.

Learning

The Endocrine System acts as the body's major chemical messenger network, working in parallel with the nervous system to maintain homeostasis and regulate long-term processes. It consists of glands like the pituitary, thyroid, adrenal, and pancreas which synthesize and secrete hormones directly into the bloodstream. These hormones act as signals, traveling to distant target cells and tissues to control vital functions such as metabolism, growth and development, sleep cycles, mood, and sexual function.

Both the endocrine system and liver are fundamental to maintaining the body's internal balance. The endocrine glands regulate hormones that control everything from stress response to metabolism, while the liver ensures proper nutrient processing, detoxification, and energy management. Together, these systems play a vital role in overall health and longevity

Chapter 51

Living well with Diabetes

Diabetes is a condition when your body either doesn't produce enough insulin or cannot use it effectively. Insulin acts like a key. It unlocks your cells allowing glucose to enter and be used for energy. Without enough insulin action, glucose stays trapped in the bloodstream, leading to high blood sugar.

Common Symptoms of Diabetes

- Increased thirst and hunger
- Frequent urination
- Fatigue or low energy
- Blurred vision
- Slow-healing wounds
- Unexplained weight loss
- Numbness or tingling in the hands or feet

What is Insulin Resistance?

The root cause of most diabetes cases is insulin resistance. This is a condition where your body's cells no longer respond properly to insulin, making it difficult for glucose to enter the cells. This causes blood sugar levels to rise.

Insulin Resistance is considered the central driver of metabolic syndrome.

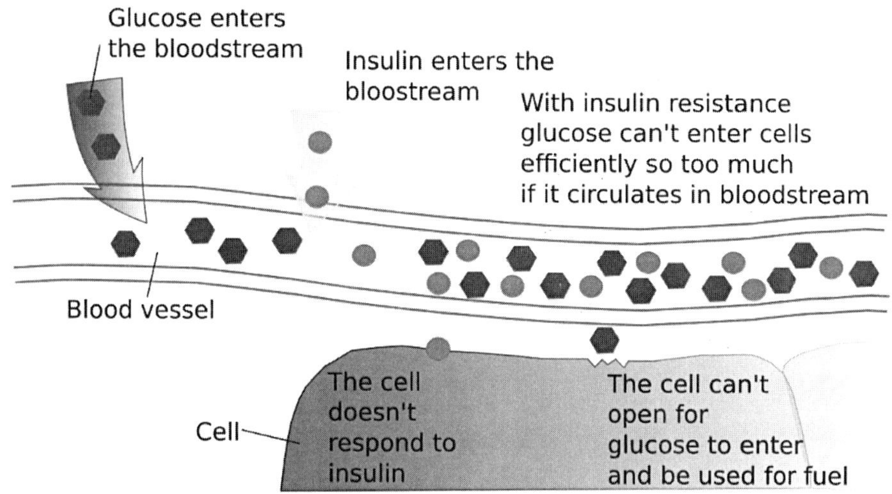

What causes Insulin Resistance?

Insulin resistance is often caused by a combination of factors:

- Belly fat and obesity
- Physical inactivity and a sedentary life style
- Poor diet (especially high intake of sugar and processed foods).
- Sleep deprivation and Chronic stress
- Genetics
- Inflammation in the body

Blood Sugar Levels

Based on guidelines from major medical associations like the American Diabetes Association (ADA), the normal levels for both Fasting Blood Sugar and Random Blood Sugar for an adult are as follows

Fasting: Less than 100 mg/dl

Random: Less than 140 mg/dl

HbA1C test:

It shows your average value of sugar over past 2–3 months

- Below 5.7% -Normal
- 5.7–6.4% -Prediabetes
- 6.5% or more- Diabetes

It is important to understand that Insulin Resistance often happens years before blood sugar levels rise. Therefore, testing insulin levels can provide an early warning sign, much before traditional glucose tests show a problem.

Long-Term Effects of Diabetes:

- If uncontrolled, diabetes can harm almost every organ and lead to:
- Heart disease and stroke
- Nerve damage (numbness, tingling)
- Kidney failure and Eye problems, even blindness
- Poor wound healing leading to Infections and amputations
- Increased risk of sleep apnea, dementia and Alzheimer's.

Prevention & Control

Diabetes is largely preventable with the right lifestyle changes. If you have prediabetes, following changes can reverse or delay its progression:

- Eat a Healthy Diet – Focus on fiber-rich and high protein foods.
- Simultaneously cut down on sugar and processed foods.
- Stay Physically Active – Aim for at least 45 minutes of moderate activity daily.

- Get rid of excess Weight – Losing just 5–10% of your body weight can significantly reduce your risk.
- Avoid prolonged sitting – Move around every 30 minutes to break up sitting time.
- Learn to manage stress to keep your body balanced

Foods for lowering blood sugar and manage diabetes

1) Leafy greens & non-starchy vegetables

These include Spinach (palak), fenugreek (methi) leaves, kale, Swiss chard, broccoli, cauliflower, asparagus, cabbage.

Reasoning: Very low in digestible carbs, high in fibre, vitamins & minerals which ae good for blood sugar.

Suggestion: Make a big portion of your plate veggies. In an Indian meal: sauté spinach with spices, make cauliflower rice, include a mixed veg curry with minimal starchy items.

2) Whole grains & legumes (instead of refined carbs. These include Oats, barley, quinoa, brown rice, millets (ragi, jowar, bajra), whole-wheat chapati; legumes (dal, chickpeas, beans, lentils).

Reasoning: These provide complex carbs + fibre, slower absorption of glucose. Good for post-meal blood sugar control.

Suggestion: Swap white rice for brown or mix half-white+half-brown rice; use millets for rotis/pancakes; include dal or beans 3–4 times a week.

3) Nuts, seeds & healthy fats

These include Almonds, walnuts, flaxseeds, chia seeds, pumpkin seeds, sesame seeds; foods like avocado if available.

Reasoning: Good fats + fibre + some protein -> help slow digestion, improve insulin sensitivity.

Suggestion: Use a small handful of nuts as a snack; sprinkle seeds in your porridge/curd; replace deep frying with light sautéing using healthy oil.

4) Lean protein & fatty fish

These include Fishes like salmon, mackerel, sardines (if accessible); lean poultry (skinless); plant-based proteins: tofu, paneer (in limited amounts), legumes.

Reasoning: Protein doesn't raise blood sugar like carbs; also useful for satiety, weight control, preserving muscle mass. Fatty fish brings omega-3s which help insulin sensitivity.

Suggestion: For Indian context: grill or bake fish/ chicken rather than deep-fry; include tofu or paneer cubes in curry with plenty of vegetables; dal+beans provide good plant protein.

5) Fruits & berries (in moderation)

These include Berries (strawberries, blueberries, raspberries) if available; guava, apple, citrus fruits; avoid juices/added sugar.

Reasoning: Although fruits contain natural sugars, those with low–moderate GI + high fibre + good nutrients are helpful rather than harmful.

Suggestion: Have fruit for snack or dessert but keep portion moderate; combine with a nut/seed or yoghurt to slow absorption.

6) Indian-style foods / spices

These include Bitter gourd (karela), fenugreek seeds (methi dana), curry leaves, Indian gooseberry (amla), turmeric/curcumin.
Reasoning: Some Indian-traditional foods/spices show promising effects for blood sugar and insulin sensitivity.

Suggestion: Example: Soak 1 teaspoon fenugreek seeds overnight and eat first thing (under dietitian supervision). Bitter gourd in a curry. Use turmeric generously in cooking.

Foods to Limit / Avoid

Refined carbs: white rice, white bread, pasta made of white flour, regular white flour chapatis without fibre.
Added sugars & sugar-sweetened beverages like sodas, sweetened juices.
Deep-fried foods, excess saturated fats, refined oils, trans-fats.
Excess portion sizes of high-GI foods.
Skipping heavy meals which have few vegetables and lots of refined carbs.

Learning

Diabetes is a serious but manageable condition. By understanding its causes, recognizing symptoms early, and adopting a healthy lifestyle, you can take charge of your health and reduce your risk of developing complications. Regularly checking blood sugar, HbA1C, and insulin levels is the key to staying ahead of this condition.

Chapter 52

Mastering your Blood Pressure

Blood Pressure is the force of blood exerted against the walls of your artery. It is denoted by two numbers:

Systolic (the denominator) is the pressure when your heart beats

Diastolic (the numerator) is the pressure when your heart rests between beats.

For example, a normal blood pressure reading is around 120/80 mmHg

Blood Pressure Ranges

Normal-Around 120/80 mm Hg

High (Hypertension) -140/90 mm Hg or more

Low (Hypotension) -Below 90/60 mm Hg (can be risky in seniors)

In the 1970s and 80s, blood pressure up to 140/90 mm Hg was often considered normal. Today, scientific evidence has shown that even mildly elevated BP can quietly damage the heart, brain, kidneys, and arteries over decades. Large long-term studies, better technology (like CT angiography and echocardiography), and improved understanding of chronic diseases revealed that the risk of heart attack and stroke rises steadily with every small increase in BP above 115 mm Hg.

As the average life span of people has now improved, these small elevations accumulate into major health problems if left untreated. Therefore, modern guidelines lowered the old "normal" range to encourage early prevention through lifestyle changes, not to promote more medicine. Most people with slightly elevated BP are advised diet, exercise, weight control, and salt reduction—not drugs.

What are the Symptoms of High Blood Pressure?

Often called the 'silent killer,' hypertension typically has no symptoms until it becomes severe. When symptoms do appear, they can include:

-Severe headaches

-Shortness of breath

-Chest pain

-Dizziness or light-headedness

-Blurred vision

-Pounding in the chest, neck, or ears

What Causes High Blood Pressure?

High blood pressure develops gradually over a period of time due to a number of factors that often work together:

1) Physical inactivity and obesity
2) Excessive alcohol consumption and smoking
3) Unhealthy diet (high salt and fat, low potassium)
4) Chronic stress
5) Genetics (family history)
6) Aging (less flexible blood vessels)

How to prevent and control Hypertension?

Hypertension can often be managed naturally with consistent life style changes:

- Get rid of excess weight. Even losing 10 kg can reduce blood pressure up to 20 points
- Exercise regularly (at least 45 minutes of moderate activity most days)
- Eat a Healthy Diet – Focus on fibre-rich and high protein foods. Simultaneously cut down on salt, sugar, saturated fats and processed foods.
- Quit smoking and avoid tobacco in all forms.
- Limit or Avoid alcohol completely.
- Manage stress: Use relaxation techniques like Yoga, Meditation which can lower BP by 5 points or more.
- Prioritize Sleep: Aim for at least 7 hours of quality sleep every night.

Foods for lowering blood pressure "naturally"

1) Leafy greens & colourful vegetables

These include: Spinach, fenugreek (methi), kale, Swiss chard, beetroot, carrots, bell peppers, okra. Vegetables (especially nitrate-rich ones like spinach, beetroot)

Reasoning: help relax/dilate blood vessels, assist in lowering blood pressure.

Suggestion: Use them generously in meals—dal with spinach, beetroot salad, stir-fried greens with garlic.

2) Fruits (especially high-potassium & antioxidant fruits)

These include: Banana, guava, papaya, orange, mango (in moderate amounts), berries (blueberries, strawberries) if available.

Reasoning: Potassium helps balance sodium effects; antioxidants reduce inflammation and vascular stress.

Suggestion: Have a fruit as snack, add fruit to your breakfast, choose whole fruit over juices.

3)Whole grains

These include: Brown rice, millet (ragi, jowar, bajra), oats, whole-wheat chapati, quinoa, barley.

Reasoning: Whole grains provide fibre, nutrients, help with cholesterol & blood pressure.

Suggestion: Swap refined flour for whole-grain flour; include at least half your grains as whole.

4) Lean proteins & especially plant-based proteins

These include: Legumes/beans (chickpeas, lentils, kidney beans), soy/edamame/tofu, fish (salmon, mackerel, sardines), skinless poultry in moderation.

Reasoning: The AHA research showed higher plant-based protein intake associated with lower hypertension risk.

Suggestion: In an Indian diet, incorporate dal + legumes 3-4 times a week; include fish or chicken 1-2 times; keep red meat minimal.

5) Nuts, seeds & healthy oils

These include: Almonds, walnuts, flaxseeds, chia seeds; use oils like olive oil, canola oil, sunflower oil (non-tropical).
Reasoning: Nuts/seeds offer healthy fats, fibre, and have been linked to improved heart/vascular health.

Suggestion: A handful of nuts as snack; use seeds sprinkled on curd/porridge; replace ghee/butter with moderate olive oil or light vegetable oil.

6) Low-fat dairy & fish high in omega-3s
These include: Low-fat milk or yogurt, curd; fish like salmon/mackerel twice a week; lean poultry.
Reasoning: Dairy with lower fat content and fatty fish help reduce heart disease risk & assist in blood pressure control.

Suggestion: Use low-fat curd in meals; grill or bake fish rather than deep-frying.

Foods to Limit / Avoid

-Sodium (salt): Keep sodium intake ideally under 1,500 mg/day, or at most ~2,300 mg/day.
-Saturated & Trans fats (full-fat dairy, fatty meats, processed meats)
-Added sugars and sugar-sweetened beverages
-Excess alcohol, ultra-processed foods, and refined grains.

Suggestions in the Indian Context

-Use dal + greens regularly (for example, dal with spinach or fenugreek) which combine plant-protein + leafy green benefits.

-Use millets (ragi, jowar, bajra) and brown rice as staples instead of mostly white rice.

-Use low-salt spice blends; avoid high-salt pickles/chips/snacks.

-Use cooking oils wisely: moderate olive oil/vegetable oil; limit ghee/butter/vanaspati.

-Snack on fruits, nuts/seeds instead of fried snacks.

-Try Indian oily fish like Surmai, Rawas, Rohu.

-When eating out, opt for grilled/steamed options, whole-grain breads/rotis where possible, avoid heavy cream-based gravies.

Innovative Scientific Ways to Reduce Blood Pressure without Medication:

1. **Slow, Controlled Breathing (Pranayama)**

This is one of the most powerful natural BP-lowering tools.

Slow breathing activates the parasympathetic (vagal) system, reduces adrenaline, relaxes blood vessels, and lowers systolic BP by 5–10 mmHg in minutes. Anulom -Vilom (Alternate Nostril Breathing), Bhramari (Bee Breath), Ujjayi and Sheetali & Sheetkari have been found very effective

2. **Isometric Handgrip Training**

This is one of the most effective methods.

Protocol:

- Hold a handgrip at 30% of your maximum force
- 2 minutes hold → 1 minute rest

- 4 cycles
- 3–4 times per week

This improves endothelial function and reduces BP by 8–12 mmHg.

3. Nitric-Oxide–Boosting Foods

These foods help relax blood vessels and improve arterial flexibility. Examples are Beetroot, Spinach, Arugula, Pomegranate, Citrus fruits, Dark chocolate (flavanols).

4. Morning Sunlight Exposure

Morning sunlight resets circadian rhythm, improves melatonin production at night, and reduces cortisol levels—leading to lower BP. 10–15 minutes of early sunlight helps regulate the autonomic nervous system.

5. Time-Restricted Eating (TRE)

Eating within an 8–10 hour window reduces insulin levels, decreases sympathetic activity, and improves arterial stiffness.

Studies show systolic BP reduction of 5–7 mmHg after 8–12 weeks of TRE.

6. Evening Walks (Post-Dinner Walks)

A 20-minute walk after dinner:

- Reduces post-meal glucose spikes
- Lowers sympathetic activation
- Helps reduce nighttime BP

7. Sauna and Heat Therapy

Regular sauna sessions:

- Improve vascular flexibility
- Reduce arterial stiffness
- Increase nitric oxide
- Reduce BP by 5–10 mmHg

Heat increases heart rate safely and improves endothelial function.

8. Reduce Artificial Light at Night (ALAN)

Artificial light at night disrupts melatonin and increases sympathetic activation, raising blood pressure.

Switching to warm, low-intensity lighting after sunset can reduce nighttime BP and improve resting levels.

9. Improve Magnesium Status (Often Overlooked)

Low magnesium increases arterial tone.

Optimize intake through: Pumpkin seeds, Almonds, Spinach, Whole grains etc. Magnesium supplementation often reduces BP by 4–6 mmHg.

10. Cold Exposure

Short exposure to mildly cold water (20–30 seconds at end of shower) improves vascular elasticity and autonomic balance.

Alternate hot–cold exposure also benefits BP.

11. Reduce Ultra-Processed Foods

UPFs increase inflammation, alter gut microbiome, and increase sodium retention.

12. Optimize Potassium and Sodium Balance

It is important to improve the sodium–potassium ratio.

Increase potassium-rich foods like Coconut water, Bananas, Sweet potatoes, Beans, Greens

Potassium helps kidneys excrete sodium and relax blood vessels.

13. Improve Sleep Duration & Quality

Poor sleep increases cortisol and sympathetic tone.

Targeting 7–8 hour sleep reduces BP by 5–10 mmHg naturally.

Key factors: Cool, dark room, Early dinner, Limited screen time before going to bed.

14. Stress-Reduction Practices That Work Quickly

Chronic stress increases adrenaline and cortisol, directly raising BP.

Proven methods:

- Meditation
- Yoga
- Pranayama
- Mindfulness
- Slow walking in nature

Even 10 minutes/day helps.

15. Weight Reduction Focused on Belly Fat

Visceral fat produces inflammatory hormones that raise BP.

Losing 5–10% of body weight can reduce systolic BP by 8–12 mmHg.

Time-restricted eating combined with walking is extremely helpful.

Learning:

Blood pressure can be reduced significantly without medication by improving autonomic balance, vascular flexibility, nitric oxide availability, circadian rhythm, and metabolic health. The most powerful combination is slow breathing, isometric handgrip training, nitric-oxide–rich foods, evening walks, sauna/heat therapy, and time-restricted eating, often producing significant BP reduction.

Chapter 53

Demystifying Cholesterol

Cholesterol is a waxy, fatty substance which is essential for various body functions. It is produced by the liver and is also found in animal-based foods which we consume. While your body needs some cholesterol, too much in the blood can significantly increase the risk of heart disease.

Sources of Cholesterol

Cholesterol is found only in animal-based foods such as meat (beef, pork, lamb), poultry (chicken, turkey), egg yolks, dairy products (milk, cheese, butter, cream), and seafood (fish, shrimp, prawns, shellfish). Plant-based foods such as fruits, vegetables, grains, nuts, and seeds contain no cholesterol.

What is the limit on consumption of dietary Cholesterol?

The liver produces all the cholesterol your body needs. There is no need to consume cholesterol-rich foods. For many years, guidelines from American Heart Association recommended limiting dietary cholesterol to less than 300 mg per day.

Good vs. Bad cholesterol

Low-Density Lipoprotein (LDL) is the "bad" cholesterol. It carries cholesterol to your blood vessels. When there is too much LDL, it builds up plaque in your in arteries, leading to heart attack and stroke.

High-Density Lipoprotein (HDL) is the "good" cholesterol. It acts like a scavenger removing excess cholesterol from the bloodstream and returns it to the liver. Higher HDL levels reduce your risk of heart disease.

Ideal Cholesterol Levels

Total cholesterol should be less than 200 mg/dL.

LDL (bad) cholesterol should be less than 100 mg/dL.

HDL (good) cholesterol should be above 60 mg/dL.

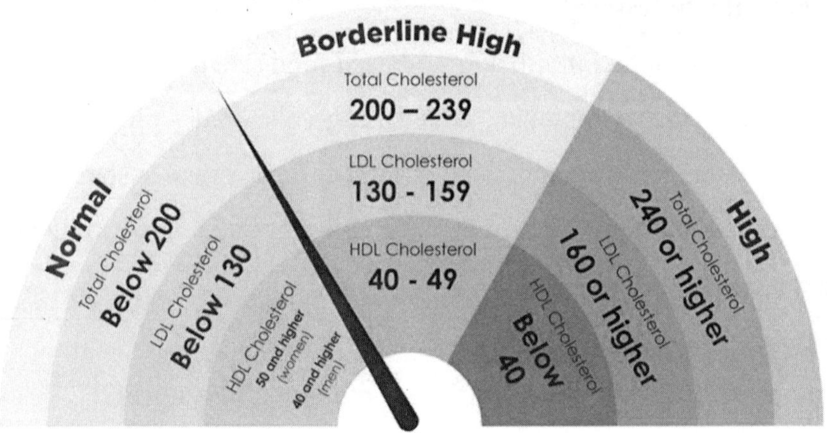

What Causes High LDL cholesterol?

High LDL is primarily caused by a lifestyle factor like a diet high in saturated fats (red meats, butter, cheese), trans fats (hydrogenated oils, processed snacks), refined carbohydrates (white bread, pastries, white rice, cookies, biscuits). Other causes include sedentary lifestyle, obesity, smoking, and genetic factors.

How Does LDL Contribute to Cardiovascular Disease?

When LDL exceeds 130 mg/dL, it leads to the formation of thick, hard plaques inside artery walls. This narrows the arteries, restricts blood flow, and raises the risk of heart attacks and strokes.

Foods to reduce your "bad" LDL cholesterol (and support overall lipid profile)

1) Soluble-fibre rich grains, legumes & vegetable which include:

- Oats porridge or rolled oats: a good breakfast option.
- Barley, millet (in Indian context) as whole grains.
- Legumes: lentils (dal), chickpeas, kidney beans.
- Vegetables like eggplant (brinjal), okra (bhindi) which are low-calorie and provide fibre.

How they help: Soluble fibre binds cholesterol and its precursors in the digestive tract, helping to remove them before they enter the bloodstream

Suggestion: Replace part of white rice with barley or millet; start breakfast with oats + fruit; include legumes 3-4 times per week.

2) Nuts, seeds & healthy oils (mono-/poly-unsaturated fats) which include:

- Nuts: almonds, walnuts (a small handful daily)
- Seeds: flaxseeds, chia seeds in porridge or curd.
- Healthy oils: olive oil (or mixed vegetable oil with good profile) instead of ghee/butter.
- Avocado (if available) for mono-unsaturated fat.

How they help: These provide healthy fats (which can improve the "good" HDL cholesterol and reduce LDL) and contain plant sterols/stanols.

Suggestion: Have 20-30 g nuts as snack; use flaxseeds mixed into your morning curd/porridge; sauté vegetables in olive oil rather than heavy ghee.

3) Fatty fish & lean animal/plant-proteins which include:

- Fatty fish: salmon, sardines, mackerel (2 to 3 servings/week)
- Lean poultry (skinless) or plant-based proteins like tofu, soy products.

How they help: Fish high in omega-3s and replacing saturated fat-rich meats helps improve lipid profile.

Suggestion: For Indian context: grilled fish or tandoori fish; if vegetarian: tofu or paneer (in moderation) + lots of vegetables.

4) Plant sterols & fortified foods which include:

- Foods fortified with plant sterols.
- Natural sources: whole grains, nuts, legumes.

How they help: Plant sterols interfere with cholesterol absorption in the intestine, lowering LDL by 5-15 %.

Suggestion: If available in your region, look for spreads/margarines enriched with plant sterols; otherwise ensure a diet rich in nuts, legumes, whole grains.

5) Fruits & vegetables rich in fibre + antioxidants which include Apples, citrus fruits, berries, Leafy greens, colourful vegetables.

How they help: Fruits/vegetables provide soluble fibre, plant-sterols, antioxidants, all help improve cholesterol profile.

Suggestion: Have 2–3 servings of fruit/day; include a large salad or vegetable side at lunch & dinner; snack on fruit instead of sweets.

6) Foods & habits to limit or avoid

-Full-fat dairy (butter, cream, full-fat cheese)

-Processed meats, red meats, sausages and fatty cuts of meat.

-Coconut oil or palm oil in excess.

How they help: Saturated fats and Trans fats raise LDL cholesterol.

Suggestion: Cook with minimal saturated fat; trim visible fat from meat; choose non-deep-fried options; use vegetable oils with good unsaturated-fat profile.

Avoid or limit these foods to lower cholesterol?

- Avoid Trans-fats in packaged snacks like namkeens, bhujia sev, chaklis, bakery items like patties, puffs, biscuits, khari, and cakes, fried street foods like samosas, bhajias, puris, batata vadas, and hydrogenated fats like vanaspati, margarine, and Dalda.
- Saturated fats to limit include ghee, butter, palm oil, coconut oil, red meat, and full-fat dairy.
- Sugary foods to avoid include Indian sweets like gulab jamun, pedha, rasgulla, jalebi, sweetened drinks like sugary chai, cold drinks, sweet lassi, packaged fruit juices, and commercial foods such as sweetened yogurts, sauces, breads, cereals, and bakery cakes.

Life style changes:

Maintain a healthy weight, exercise regularly through brisk walking, yoga, swimming, jogging, or strength training. Manage stress and get quality sleep.

Learning

The liver produces all the cholesterol your body needs, which is why dietary cholesterol from foods has less impact on blood levels. The problem arises with LDL that transports it and causes plaque buildup in arteries. HDL acts like a scavenger, removing excess cholesterol and returning it to the liver for disposal. High levels of saturated and trans fats in the diet are the primary culprits that raise unhealthy LDL levels. Cholesterol is vital for body but its levels must be maintained within limits. Choose healthy fats and whole foods. Avoid trans fats, excess saturated fats, and sugar. Be physically active and maintain a healthy lifestyle

Chapter 54
All about Heart Blockages

The term heart blockage can mean two different things. It can be a physical blockage in your arteries (atherosclerosis) or a problem with your heart's electrical signals.

Coronary Artery Blockage (Atherosclerosis)

This refers to the clogging of the coronary arteries — the tubes that supply oxygen-rich blood to the heart muscle. Over a period of time, a sticky substance called plaque (made up of fat, cholesterol, calcium, and other substances) builds up on the inner walls of these tubes. This narrows them and restricts blood flow. This condition is commonly known as coronary artery disease.

How it develops?

- Plaque Formation: Fatty deposits accumulate along artery walls.
- Narrowing of Arteries: The buildup reduces blood flow to the heart.
- Blood Clots: A ruptured plaques may form a blood clot, causing sudden blockages and a heart attack.

Common Symptoms

- Chest pain (Angina) – especially during exertion or stress
- Shortness of breath
- Fatigue

- Heart attack symptoms: Severe chest pain, sweating, nausea, pain radiating to the arm, jaw, or back

Non-invasive Cardiac CT Angiography

Cardiac CT Angiography has rapidly become one of the most important tools for evaluating heart health—especially for detecting blockages in the coronary arteries. It is non-invasive, quick, and highly precise. A treadmill test or echo test may appear normal even with 30–50% blockages, but CCTA will show them clearly.

Benefit of Cardiac CT Angiography

A. Non-invasive and extremely safe

- No catheter inserted into the arteries
- No hospitalization needed
- Very low risk compared to conventional angiography
- Completed in 5–10 minutes

B. Exceptional diagnostic accuracy

C. Provides extra information beyond blockages like Heart size and pumping function, Aortic and lung structures, Coronary calcium score etc.

D. Ideal for preventive health check-up.

It is currently the best first-line diagnostic tool for most patients with suspected coronary artery disease, and the best preventive screening tool for those with risk factors, family history, or lifestyle concerns.

Degrees of Heart Blockages:

1) Minor Blockages

Minor blockages (less than 20–30%) are common and usually without symptoms.

2) Moderate Blockage (50% Blockage)

It means that half the artery's diameter is obstructed by plaque. Often, there are no symptoms at rest, but angina or breathlessness during activity may occur.

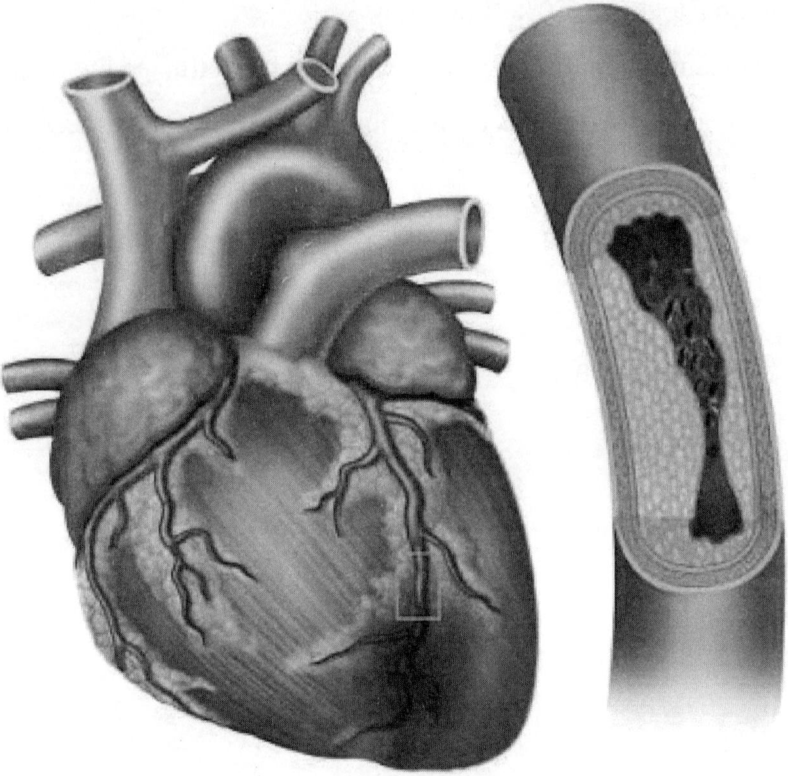

Normal Artery

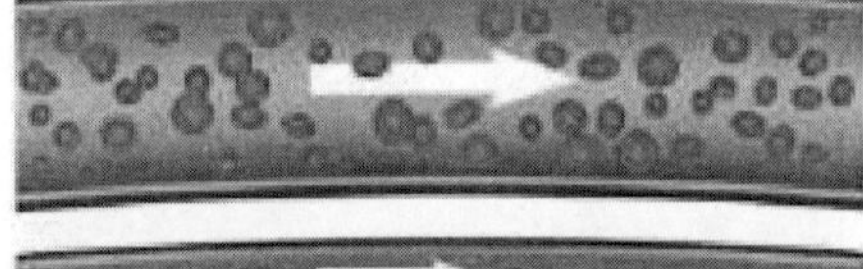

Partial Block

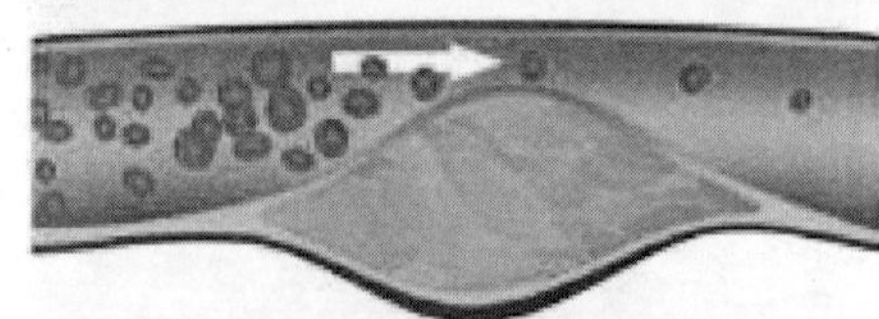

Complete Block

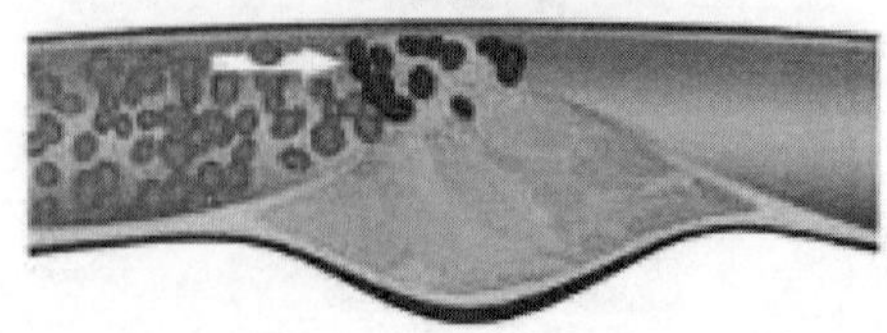

Management:

- Lifestyle changes (diet, exercise, quit smoking)
- Medications (blood thinners, statins, and nitrates)
- Regular medical check-ups

3) Severe Blockage (80–90% Blockage)

It means that a large portion of the artery is blocked, severely limiting blood flow.

Symptoms:

- Angina even at rest
- Shortness of breath, fatigue, dizziness
- High risk of heart attack

Management:

- Angioplasty with Stenting
- Coronary Artery Bypass.
- Medications to manage cholesterol, prevent clots, and support heart function

When is Intervention Required?

Moderate Blockage: Usually managed with medications and lifestyle changes.

Severe Blockage: Often requires urgent medical or surgical intervention.

Can Heart Block Be Prevented?

While not all heart blocks are preventable, you can significantly reduce your risk with a heart-healthy lifestyle:

- Eat a nutritious, low-fat, low-sodium diet
- Exercise regularly

- Avoid smoking and limit alcohol
- Manage stress through yoga, meditation, or hobbies
- Maintain a healthy weight
- Ensure 7–8 hours of quality sleep
- Schedule routine heart health check-ups

Electrical Heart Blocks (Arrhythmia)

The heart beats through a carefully timed electrical system. Heart block occurs when these signals are delayed or blocked from reaching the lower chambers of the heart, leading to a slow or irregular heartbeat. Arrhythmia can be detected with an ECG.

What is a peacemaker and what it does?

A pacemaker is a crucial medical device used to treat various heart rhythm disorders known as arrhythmias. When the heart's natural electrical system isn't working correctly, it acts as an artificial substitute ensuring that the heart continues to beat regularly and effectively to pump blood throughout the body.

How Blockages Cause a Heart Attack

A heart attack (Myocardial Infarction) is fundamentally caused by the rupture of an existing blockage in a coronary artery. The blockage itself is a buildup of fatty plaque that narrows the artery and reduces blood flow. When this plaque ruptures, the body triggers the formation of a blood clot on the rupture. This sudden blood clot then acts as a complete or severe plug, totally cutting off the supply of oxygen-rich blood to the section of the heart muscle fed by that artery. Because heart muscle cells cannot survive long without oxygen, this lack of blood flow causes the affected tissue to die, resulting in the acute event known as a heart attack.

Learning:

Whether it is arterial blockage or electrical heart block, early detection and management can make a huge difference in outcomes. Listen to your body signals and consult your doctor if you experience any warning signs.

Chapter 55

Myths of BP, Diabetes & Cholesterol

It is extremely important to separate facts from misconceptions. Despite decades of research, several myths continue to mislead people, causing fear, wrong treatment choices, and avoidable health risks. Understanding what is true and what is not can enable individuals to take informed steps toward better health.

"If I Feel Fine, My BP/Cholesterol/Sugar Must Be Normal."

Fact: All three conditions are called "silent killers" for a reason. High BP usually has no symptoms. High cholesterol causes no early warning signs. Type 2 diabetes may remain silent for years before diagnosis. Regular testing is the only way to know your numbers.

"Medicines Are Harmful; I Should Avoid Them as Long as Possible."

Fact: Medicines for BP, cholesterol (statins), and diabetes are among the most researched and safest when used correctly. They prevent heart attacks, strokes, kidney failure, and nerve damage. Delaying medicines when they are needed allows silent damage to progress. Lifestyle changes are essential but often work best when combined with medication.

"Once I Start Medicines, I Must Take Them for Life."

Fact: Not always.

For many people, sustained weight loss, regular exercise, and dietary changes can reduce BP normalize cholesterol and improve sugar control. Some individuals can reduce dosage or stop medicines under medical supervision. The key is consistent lifestyle improvement, not sudden withdrawal.

"Only Fat or Obese People Get Diabetes or High BP."

Fact: While weight is a major risk factor, thin people can also develop diabetes, high BP, or high cholesterol, especially if they eat high-sugar or high-fat foods, have genetics that predispose them, lead sedentary lives, have high stress or poor sleep. Metabolic health matters more than body size alone.

"Sugar causes Diabetes."

Fact: Eating sugar alone does not directly cause diabetes, but excess sugar leads to Weight gain, Insulin resistance and Fatty liver. These conditions increase the risk of type 2 diabetes. It is not sugar alone—total lifestyle and calorie excess are responsible.

"I Don't Eat Much Salt, so I won't get high BP"

Fact: Excess salt is a major factor, but not the only one. Other important contributors include, stress and poor sleep, sedentary lifestyle, excess weight, alcohol, high sodium in packaged foods (even if food does not taste salty). BP control requires a holistic approach, not just low salt.

"Walking daily is enough to Control All Three Conditions."

Fact: Walking is very good but not enough by itself. Walking should be part of a bigger lifestyle routine. Effective control requires, strength training, aerobic exercise, weight management, better sleep, reduced stress and smart nutrition

"BP, Cholesterol, and Diabetes Are Separate Problems."

Fact: They are deeply connected. Together they accelerate artery damage, heart attacks, strokes, kidney disease. Managing them together is the best protection for long-term health.

"All Cholesterol Is Bad."

Fact: Cholesterol is essential for hormones, cell membranes, and vitamin D production.

The problem is high LDL ('bad' cholesterol) and low HDL ('good' cholesterol).

Not all cholesterol is harmful—only the imbalanced levels are.

"Brown Sugar, Jaggery, and Honey Are Better for Diabetes."

Fact: They are not healthier options for diabetics.

All raise blood glucose almost equally.

"Diabetes means giving up all Carbs."

Fact: Carbs are essential. The objective should be to choose complex hydrocarbons like whole grains, high-fibre vegetables, legumes, millets etc. At the same time, it is necessary to avoid or limit white rice, white bread, sugary snacks, refined flour foods

“Heart Attacks Only Happen If Cholesterol Is Very High.”

Fact: Heart attacks often occur even when cholesterol is “border-line.” The real culprits could be high BP, high sugar, high LDL, inflammation, smoking or stress

“Diabetes Is Inevitable If It Runs in the Family.”

Fact: Genes contribute, but lifestyle determines expression.

With healthy habits, many people with strong family history never develop diabetes.

“High BP, Cholesterol, and Diabetes Are Only for Older People.”

Fact: These conditions increasingly affect younger adults—even those in their 20s and 30s. Sedentary lifestyle, high stress, poor sleep, processed foods, and obesity are major contributors. Early detection is crucial because damage to blood vessels begins long before symptoms appear.

Learning:

BP, cholesterol, and diabetes are manageable and often preventable. Myths create unnecessary fear and lead to poor decisions. Evidence-based lifestyle habits, combined with periodic testing and timely medication, offer the best protection for a long, healthy, and active life.

Chapter 56

Haemoglobin: The Lifeline of your Blood

Haemoglobin is an iron-rich protein found in red blood cells. It plays a vital role in transporting oxygen from the lungs to every cell in the body and carrying carbon dioxide back to the lungs for exhalation. It gives blood its characteristic red colour and is essential for maintaining energy and vitality.

Where is Haemoglobin Produced?

Haemoglobin is produced in the bone marrow—the soft, spongy tissue inside bones where new red blood cells are formed.

Functions of Haemoglobin

1. Oxygen Transport: Binds with oxygen in the lungs and delivers it to tissues and organs throughout the body.
2. Carbon Dioxide Removal: Collects carbon dioxide from tissues and transports it to the lungs for elimination.

Normal Haemoglobin Levels

- Men: 14 – 18 g/dL
- Women: 12 – 16 g/dL

Why Are Healthy Haemoglobin Levels Important?

Maintaining adequate haemoglobin levels is crucial for the body's proper functioning. Low haemoglobin can lead to fatigue, dizziness, pale skin, poor concentration, and even organ damage in severe cases. It may also result in anaemia, reducing the blood's capacity to carry oxygen.

Causes of Low Haemoglobin

- Poor nutrition
- Blood loss (injury, menstruation, surgery)
- Chronic diseases (kidney disease, cancer)
- Bone marrow disorders
- Side effects of certain medications or cancer treatments

Ways to Naturally Boost Haemoglobin Levels

Ensure that your daily diet includes the following:

1. Iron-Rich Foods

Iron is the key building block of haemoglobin.

- Animal Sources: Red meat, liver, poultry, fish, clams, and oysters
- Plant Sources: Leafy greens (spinach, kale), lentils, beans, soybeans, tofu, pumpkin seeds, sesame seeds, cashews, and fortified cereals

2. Vitamin C

Vitamin C helps your body absorb iron more efficiently. Add these to your meals:

- Citrus fruits (oranges, lemons, grapefruits)
- Berries (strawberries, blueberries)
- Tomatoes, bell peppers, broccoli, kiwi, mango, papaya

3. Folate (Vitamin B9)

Folate is essential for the production of healthy red blood cells:

- Leafy greens (spinach, romaine lettuce)

- Legumes (lentils, beans, peas)
- Citrus fruits, avocados, broccoli
- Fortified grains

4. Vitamin B12

Vitamin B12 supports the production of RBCs and prevents anaemia:

- Meat, poultry, fish (salmon, tuna, sardines)
- Dairy (milk, yogurt, cheese)
- Eggs
- Fortified plant-based milks and nutritional yeast

5. Vitamin B6

Vitamin B6 helps in haemoglobin production:

- Chicken, pork, fish
- Spinach, bell peppers, potatoes
- Chickpeas, lentils, soybeans
- Nuts and seeds (sunflower, peanuts, hazelnuts)

6. Copper

Copper aids iron absorption:

- Liver, shellfish
- Nuts and seeds (cashews, sesame seeds)
- Legumes, whole grains

7. Stay Hydrated

Drinking 8–10 glasses of water daily supports healthy blood volume and circulation, which aids red blood cell production.

8. Exercise Regularly

Physical activity boosts red blood cell production. Aim to include:

- Brisk walking or jogging
- Yoga and strength training
- Cycling or swimming

Recommended Daily Intake of Supplements:

• Iron: 20 mg

• Vitamin B6: 50 mg

• Folic Acid (B9): 500 mcg

• Vitamin B12: 1500 mcg

• Vitamin C: 1000 mg

Learning:

Boosting your haemoglobin naturally is very much achievable through mindful eating, proper hydration and regular physical activity. A balanced diet rich in iron, vitamin C, folate, B12, and B6 is the foundation. Healthy haemoglobin means a healthier, more energetic body.

Chapter 57

Lifestyle Diseases – A curse of the Modern Age

Rapid technological advances, unrealistic ambitions, demanding work responsibility, stiff competition, and lack of time have brought about major changes in the way we lead our life causing a number of chronic diseases.

Lifestyle diseases are health conditions primarily caused by a person's daily habits and way of living. These illnesses develop slowly over time due to unhealthy diet, lack of physical activity, chronic stress, smoking, alcohol consumption, and inadequate sleep. They are on the rise globally, affecting people of all ages, and are now among the leading causes of death and disability.

Metabolic Syndrome – The Silent Alarm

One of the most serious consequences of poor lifestyle choices is metabolic syndrome. This is a cluster of health risks that significantly increase your chance of developing serious conditions like diabetes, heart disease, and stroke.

A diagnosis of metabolic syndrome is made when at least three of the following five risk factors are present:

1. High blood pressure (greater than 130/85)
2. Elevated fasting glucose (greater than 110)
3. Excess abdominal fat (waist circumference > 40 inches for men, > 35 inches for women)

4. Low HDL cholesterol levels (less than 40 mg/dL)
5. High triglycerides (greater than 150 mg/dL)

The underlying causes are rooted in lifestyle choices, especially insulin resistance, obesity, and a sedentary lifestyle.

Causes of Lifestyle Diseases

These diseases are driven by a combination of unhealthy choices and modern-day living. Main causes are as follows:

-*Unhealthy Diet*: A diet high in sugar, salt, and saturated fats and low in fruits, vegetables, and fibre can lead to obesity, high cholesterol, and blood sugar issues. Overeating and frequent consumption of processed foods are also major culprits.

-*Physical Inactivity*: A sedentary lifestyle (e.g., long hours of sitting) reduces calorie burning and weakens muscle tone, increasing the risk of obesity, cardiovascular disease, type 2 diabetes, and certain cancers.

-*Tobacco Use*: Smoking or chewing tobacco is directly linked to heart disease, stroke, chronic respiratory diseases, and various cancers. Even passive smoking is harmful.

-*Alcohol Consumption*: Excessive alcohol damages the liver, heart, pancreas, and brain, raising the risk of high blood pressure, stroke, obesity, and several cancers.

-*Chronic Stress*: Long-term stress triggers hormonal imbalances and inflammation, which are linked to heart disease, hypertension, digestive problems, depression, and sleep disorders.

-*Lack of Quality Sleep*: Poor sleep hygiene or sleep disorders (like insomnia or sleep apnea) increase the risk of obesity, diabetes, and heart disease.

-*Genetic Predisposition*: While lifestyle is key, a family history of conditions like diabetes or heart disease can combine with poor habits to accelerate disease onset.

Common Lifestyle Diseases:

-Cardiovascular Diseases: High blood pressure, heart attacks, and strokes.

-Type-2 Diabetes and Obesity.

-Cancers, especially those linked to smoking (e.g., lung) or diet.

-Chronic Respiratory Diseases: Asthma and COPD (chronic obstructive pulmonary disease).

-Liver Disease (including fatty liver).

-Kidney Disease and Osteoporosis.

-Mental Health Disorders: Depression, anxiety, and insomnia.

-Neurodegenerative Diseases: Alzheimer’s and Parkinson’s.

Triggers and the Lifestyle Diseases caused

Each unhealthy habit contributes to specific health problems:

-*Stress*: Elevates blood pressure, increases heart rate, and can cause anxiety, depression, and digestive issues like irritable bowel syndrome (IBS).

-*Excess Sugar*: Leads to insulin resistance (the pathway to type 2 diabetes), promotes obesity, and contributes to inflammation, which harms the heart.

-*Unhealthy Fats*: Saturated and trans fats raise "bad" cholesterol (LDL) and lower "good" cholesterol (HDL), promoting heart disease, obesity, and worsening insulin resistance.

-*Salt*: The primary dietary cause of high blood pressure, which strains the heart and kidneys.

When these factors are combined—stress, sugar, fat, and salt—they amplify each other's harmful effects, making lifestyle diseases even more likely.

How to Prevent Lifestyle Diseases?

Lifestyle diseases arise from long-term disruptions in metabolic, hormonal, inflammatory, and autonomic systems. Scientific evidence shows that 80–90% of these conditions are preventable through appropriate lifestyle changes. Prevention requires holistic, science-backed strategies to prevent lifestyle diseases.

1. Optimal Nutrition:

Nutrition is the Foundation of Metabolic Health. Diet has a direct influence on glucose regulation, lipid metabolism, inflammation, gut microbiota, and oxidative stress—all key determinants of chronic disease.

Eat only Whole, Unprocessed Foods. Whole foods provide fibre, phytonutrients, antioxidants, minerals, and vitamins that regulate Insulin sensitivity, Gut microbial diversity, chronic inflammation and Oxidative stress

High-fibre carbohydrates (whole grains, fruits, vegetables) slow glucose absorption and stabilise postprandial spikes.

Lean proteins (pulses, dairy, eggs, fish, and soy) increase satiety, preserve lean mass, and support metabolic rate.

Unsaturated fats (omega-3s, MUFAs, PUFAs) lower LDL-C, reduce triglycerides, and improve endothelial function.

Limit Harmful foods like Added sugars, Trans fats, Excess sodium, Ultra-processed foods.

2. Body Weight and Visceral Fat:

Excess adipose tissue—particularly visceral fat impairs insulin signalling and cause metabolic dysfunction.

A 5–10% weight reduction improves insulin sensitivity, reduces hepatic steatosis, lowers blood pressure, and normalises triglycerides.

Waist circumference is a better predictor of disease risk than BMI because it reflects visceral fat burden.

How to Reduce Adiposity

- Calorie deficit from diet and increased activity.
- Higher protein intake to maintain muscle mass.
- Adequate sleep to stabilise ghrelin and leptin.
- Stress reduction to limit cortisol-induced fat deposition.

3. Physical Activity: The Most Potent Intervention

Physical activity improves nearly every biomarker related to chronic disease.

-Improves glucose uptake and reversing insulin resistance.

-Enhances cellular energy efficiency.

-Reduces systemic inflammation and oxidative stress.

-Improves nitric oxide availability.

-Preserves lean muscle mass, preventing sarcopenia and metabolic slowdown.

Exercise at least sixty minutes per day to incorporate moderate aerobic activity, Strength training at least 2–3 days/week to enhance muscle mass and metabolic rate, reduce sedentary time, as sitting more than 8 hours/day increases cardiovascular risk.

4. Sleep: Hormonal Regulation and Metabolic Reset

Sleep deprivation alters multiple systems linked to lifestyle diseases.

-Increases cortisol, elevating BP and blood glucose.

-Reduces insulin sensitivity by 20–30%.

-Elevates inflammatory markers (CRP).

-Target 7–8 hours of restorative sleep/day, Consistent circadian rhythm,

-Screen-free wind-down routine to protect melatonin release.

5. Stress and Neurohormonal Balance

Chronic stress leads to:

- Persistent cortisol secretion
- Elevated blood glucose
- Increased visceral adiposity
- Hypertension
- Reduced immunity

Managing Stress

Mindfulness meditation reduces amygdala activation and sympathetic drive.

Yoga and pranayama enhance vagal tone and reduce inflammatory signalling.

Nature exposure increases parasympathetic activity and reduces cortisol.

6. Avoiding Tobacco and Moderating Alcohol

Tobacco

- Damages endothelium, promotes plaque formation.
- Causes oxidative stress and inflammation.
- Increases cancer, stroke, and heart attack risk.

Alcohol

- Excess intake causes fatty liver, hypertension, arrhythmias, and cancers.
- Even moderate drinking increases breast and colon cancer risk.
- Abstinence or very limited consumption is scientifically safest.

7. Regular Health Screening: Early Detection and Prevention

Screening identifies subclinical abnormalities before symptoms appear:

Key Tests

- Blood pressure
- Fasting glucose, OGTT, HbA1c
- Lipid profile
- Liver and kidney function tests
- Thyroid function
- Vitamin D and B12
- hs-CRP for inflammation
- ECG/Echo after 45 or earlier if high risk

Early intervention prevents escalation to full-blown disease.

8. Gut Microbiome Health

A healthy gut is now seen as central to overall metabolic wellness. Emerging science shows that gut microbial diversity is linked to Lower inflammation, Better glucose metabolism, Improved lipid regulation and Stronger immunity.

How to Strengthen the Microbiome

- High-fibre diet (prebiotics)
- Fermented foods (probiotics)
- Reduced antibiotics and processed foods
- Polyphenol-rich foods (turmeric, berries, herbs, spices)

Scientific literature conclusively shows that when these pillars are addressed, chronic disease risk can be reduced by 70–90%, and biological ageing slows significantly.

Learning:

Lifestyle diseases are often a byproduct of modern living. However, Science has shown us how to prevent them. By changing our habits and adopting healthy life style, we can take control of our health. Lifestyle is not just behaviour; it is a therapeutic tool, a biological modifier, and the most powerful prescription for lifelong health.

Chapter 58

Stress- The Giant Killer

Stress is an inescapable part of modern life. It's the body's natural response to a change in the environment. We feel a jolt of stress when crossing a busy street or before a job interview. This kind of acute stress is normal and helps us stay alert and focused in difficult situations. However, stress becomes problematic when we remain under its influence for long periods. This chronic stress exhausts our system and makes us susceptible to severe health problems.

Stressors of the Primitive era and the Modern Era

Stresses of Primitive Era: The primary stressors revolved around immediate survival. The constant threat of being hunted by wild animals, finding enough food and water, and surviving natural disasters were daily struggles.

Stressors of Modern Era: In today's fast-paced world, the sources of stress have changed completely. Chronic stressors now include concerns about job security, debt, and the cost of living. Demanding workloads, difficult bosses, academic pressure, and the "rat race" to get ahead can all cause sustained stress, which leads to serious effects on our mental, emotional, and physical health.

Acute vs. Chronic Stress

- Acute (Short-Term) Stress: This is the body's immediate response to a demanding or dangerous situation. The body recovers quickly from it once the stressor is gone.
- Chronic (Long-Term) Stress: This is caused by stressful situations or events that last for a prolonged period, such as a difficult job or a long-term family problem. Chronic stress can cause serious health issues.

The Body's Stress Response: "Fight or Flight"

When faced with a perceived threat, your body goes through rapid changes to prepare you to either confront the danger or escape it. The brain's hypothalamus detects the threat and activates the sympathetic nervous system. This triggers a rush of hormones like adrenaline and cortisol, which makes your heart beat faster, your breathing quicken, and your muscles tense. All these changes prepare you to bravely face the challenge ("fight") or quickly get away from it ("flight").

When the threat is gone, the body initiates a return to its baseline state through the parasympathetic nervous system, often called the "rest and digest" system. This system counteracts the effects of "fight or flight"—your heart rate and blood pressure decrease, your breathing slows, and your muscles relax. In essence, your body returns to a state of calm and equilibrium.

HOW STRESS AFFECTS THE BODY

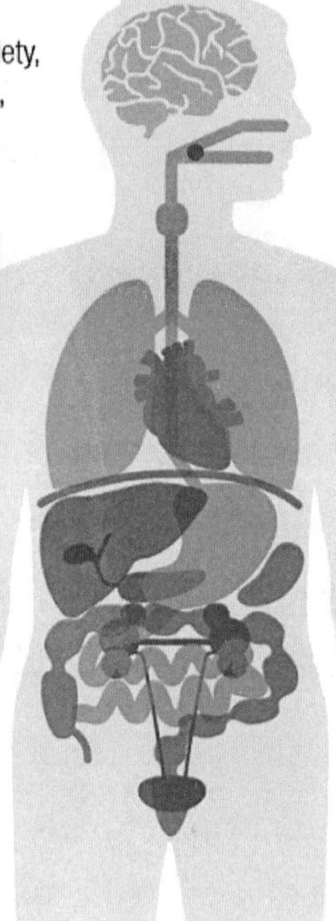

BRAIN
Difficulty concentrating, anxiety, depression, irritability, mood, mind fog

CARDIOVASCULAR
higher cholesterol, high blood pressure, increased risk of heart attack and stroke

JOINTS AND MUSCLES
increased inflammation, tension, aches and pains, muscle tightness

IMMUNE SYSTEM
decreased immune function, lowered immune defenses, increased risk of becoming ill, increase in recovery time

SKIN
hair loss, dull/brittle hair, brittle nails, dry skin, acne, delayed tissue repair

GUT
nutrient absorption, diarrhea, constipation, indigestion, bloating, pain and discomfort

REPRODUCTIVE SYSTEM
decreased hormone production, decrease in libido, increase in PMS symptoms

How stress silently amplifies Disease?

Chronic stress is a major contributor to many health conditions because of the following reasons:

-Increases blood pressure and inflammation, raising the risk of heart disease.

-Elevates blood sugar and promotes insulin resistance.

-Increases the risk of anxiety, depression, Alzheimer’s, and Parkinson’s.

-Leads to chronic muscle pain, poor posture, and spinal issues.
-Weakens your immune system.
-Is linked to the onset of autoimmune diseases.

How to Combat Stress

Stress has become an unavoidable part of modern life. While short bursts of stress can sharpen focus and improve performance, chronic stress, the type that persists day after day, can damage nearly every system in the body. It elevates cortisol and adrenaline, disrupts sleep, increases blood pressure, weakens immunity, disturbs digestion, alters mood, and accelerates ageing.

Fortunately, stress is not only manageable, it is reversible. With the right tools, we can train the mind and body to stay balanced even in demanding situations. Science shows that stress reduction is one of the most powerful ways to improve overall health and prevent lifestyle diseases.

1. Understand What Stress Really Is

Stress is a physiological and psychological response to perceived threats or challenges. When the brain senses danger, the hypothalamus activates the sympathetic nervous system and the HPA axis, releasing stress hormones (cortisol, adrenaline, noradrenaline).
While useful in emergencies, chronic activation leads to:

- high BP and heart rate
- insulin resistance
- inflammation

- muscle tension
- anxiety and irritability
- hormonal imbalance
- weakened immunity

Understanding this mechanism helps us appreciate why managing stress is vital for long-term well-being.

2. Practise Deep Breathing and Pranayama

The fastest way to calm the mind is through the breath. Deep breathing stimulates the vagus nerve, activating the parasympathetic system, which counters the stress response.

Effective Techniques are Diaphragmatic breathing, (a slow, deep belly breaths), Alternate nostril breathing (Anulom-Vilom) which balances both brain hemispheres, Bhramari pranayama – humming sound reduces anxiety rapidly.

Just 5–10 minutes daily lowers cortisol, slows the heart rate, and induces a sense of inner stability.

3. Adopt a Regular Exercise Routine

Physical activity is one of the most scientifically proven stress relievers.

How Exercise Reduces Stress

- Increases endorphins, the body's natural mood elevators.
- Enhances production of serotonin and dopamine.
- Reduces cortisol levels.
- Improves sleep and energy levels.
- Breaks the cycle of rumination and worry.

Best Options are Brisk walking, Jogging, Cycling, Yoga, Strength training, Dancing and Swimming

Even a 20-minute walk can dramatically improve mental well-being.

4. Improve Sleep Quality

Poor sleep magnifies stress, and stress disrupts sleep—a vicious cycle.

Sleep Practices That Help

- Maintain a fixed sleep schedule.
- Avoid screens 1–2 hours before bed.
- Keep the bedroom cool, dark, and quiet.
- Avoid caffeine after 4 pm.
- Practise relaxation breathing before bedtime.

Restorative sleep reduces cortisol, improves emotional resilience, and sharpens memory and focus.

5. Nourish the Body Wisely

Certain foods can increase stress (sugars, caffeine, processed foods), while others support a calm nervous system.

Diet for Stress Reduction

- Complex carbohydrates for steady glucose supply.
- Omega-3 fats (flaxseeds, walnuts, fish) to reduce inflammation and anxiety.
- Magnesium-rich foods (spinach, nuts, seeds) to relax muscles.
- Vitamin B-rich foods (whole grains, eggs, legumes) for neurotransmitter balance.
- Herbs: Ashwagandha, chamomile, holy basil help lower stress hormones.

A balanced diet keeps the mind stable and energy levels consistent throughout the day.

6. Practise Mindfulness and Meditation

Mindfulness trains the brain to stay in the present moment. Numerous studies show it reduces activity in the brain's fear centre and strengthens regions responsible for emotional control.

Effective Approaches

- 10–15 minutes of silent meditation.
- Guided meditation apps.
- Body-scan relaxation.
- Mindful walking.
- Gratitude journaling.

These practices cultivate inner peace and reduce unnecessary mental chatter.

7. Strengthen Social Connections

Good relations with friends and family influence our outlook. Strong relationships act as a powerful buffer against stress.

Benefits

- Talking with trusted people reduces anxiety.
- Shared experiences enhance emotional security.
- Laughter increases endorphins.
- Support systems help in problem-solving.

Regular interaction with family, friends, colleagues, or community groups makes daily challenges easier to handle.

8. Manage Time and Expectations

Much stress arises from overcommitment. Learn to say "no" without guilt.

- Prioritise essential tasks.
- Break big tasks into smaller steps.
- Avoid multitasking.
- Schedule short breaks during long work sessions.

Effective time management creates room for rest and recovery.

9. Reduce Digital Overload

Excess screen time, constant notifications, and social media comparisons increase stress significantly.

Digital Hygiene

- Set specific times for checking messages.
- Keep the phone away during meals, meetings, and bedtime.
- Limit exposure to negative news.
- Create "screen-free zones" at home.

A quieter digital environment calms the mind.

Some proactive ways to counter Stress

Stress is inevitable, but learning to manage it is crucial. A combination of mental, physical and lifestyle strategies can significantly reduce its impact.

-Often what we fear does not happen. Cultivate realistic optimism and prepare the mind to face the worst situation that may arise.
-Stress often comes from worrying about the future or feeling guilty about the past. Plan reasonably achievable goals within the framework of the day and completely focus only on those targets. This prevents the mind from being "wasted" in another time zone past or future. If you want peace of mind, shut the gate behind you, so that your worries are left behind. Do not touch the past – for remember, the past is dead and gone.
-Control Your Attitude. Recognize that while external situations can get out of hand, your attitude is always within your control.
-Understand your own strengths and weaknesses. Develop inner strength through self-awareness, adaptability and flexibility
-Build a daily Mindfulness practice. Mindfulness trains your brain to stay in the present moment, reducing anxiety about the future.
-Cultivate Gratitude and practice Forgiveness
-Exercise daily. Physical activity releases endorphins—your brain's natural stress relievers. Choose and do what you enjoy like, jogging, brisk walking, Yoga or dancing.

Learning:

Stress is an inevitable part of life, but suffering from it is not. By understanding its biological roots and adopting proven techniques—breathing practices, exercise, sleep optimization, mindful living, balanced nutrition, social support, and good time management—we can effectively regulate the stress response.

The goal is not to eliminate stress, but to strengthen resilience, so the mind remains calm and the body remains healthy even when life becomes challenging.

With consistent practice, anyone can transform stress into strength and live with greater clarity, balance, and joy.

Section 5
Navigating Life in the Modern Age

Chapter 59

Live longer and stay fit till the last day of Life

The desire to live a long, healthy, and active life is universal. The advancements in medical science and lifestyle awareness are supporting us to fulfil this desire.

Understanding the Aging Process

Aging is a complex biological process. Every day, billions of cells in our body die and are replaced by new ones. However, as we grow older, our ability to regenerate cells weakens. External factors like free radicals, UV radiation, and environmental toxins further accelerate this decline by damaging cells. While aging cannot be stopped entirely, science shows that we can certainly slow it down by following a healthy lifestyle

Age old observations about Living a Long and Healthy Life

-Reaching your 60s with minimal health issues improves your odds of living up to 100.

-After 70, take precautions to prevent falls, accidents and bed rest beyond three days due to illness.

-Keep moving daily. Cultivate purpose and joy

-Have strong relations with family and friends.

The last decade has seen remarkable advances in longevity research, neuroscience, nutrition, genetics, and preventive medicine. This has given us a clearer understanding of the process of Ageing and secrets of Longevity. Living merely a long life is no longer a goal. Modern science now aims for something far more meaningful- living long while staying strong, sharp, mobile, and free of disease, right till the final day.

Recommendations of Modern Science for Longevity & Fitness

As per modern science, the core pillars of lifelong health and vitality can be summarised as follows:

1. Move Daily: The Best Longevity Pill

Exercise is universally accepted as the most potent intervention for living longer and staying functional. Just 60 minutes per day can cut mortality risk by 30–40%. It supports Heart and lung health, metabolic and hormonal balance, insulin sensitivity, Muscle mass and bone strength (prevents frailty). Brain function, memory, mood lift, and gives protection against neurodegenerative diseases.

The Most Important Forms of Exercise for Longevity:

- Zone 2 Aerobic Training: (Brisk walk, cycling, swimming) for sustained cardiorespiratory health.
- Strength Training: (2–3 times weekly) to maintain muscle mass and bone density, preventing frailty.
- VO_2 Max Training: (Short bursts of high intensity) for cardiovascular performance.
- Flexibility & Balance: (Yoga, Tai Chi) to prevent falls and maintain mobility.

2. Nutrition: Eat Smart

Good nutrition is the foundation of lifelong health. Modern research shows that food is not just fuel—it is information that instructs our cells how to age.

- Prioritize Whole Foods: Eat mostly whole, minimally processed foods.
- Protein is Paramount: Prioritize protein (1.0–1.5 g per kg of weight) to maintain muscles and counter age-related loss (sarcopenia).
- Load Up on Micronutrients: Fill your plate with vegetables and fruits for antioxidants and fibre.
- Choose Healthy Fats: Incorporate olive oil, nuts, seeds, and Omega-3 rich fish.
- Avoid Overeating: Caloric excess accelerates aging; consider time-restricted eating (10–12 hour eating window).

3. Metabolism: Maintain Strong Muscles and Bones

After the age of 40, we naturally lose muscle and bone every year. Experts call muscle the true organ of longevity. Loss of muscle mass is the root cause of frailty and loss of independence.

- Focus on Strength Training: At least 2–3 times weekly.
- Optimize Intake: Ensure adequate Vitamin D, Calcium, B12, and Omega-3s.
- Prevent Falls: Practice balance training (e.g., Tai Chi or yoga).

4. Manage Weight and Waist Circumference

Abdominal fat is recognized as an active inflammatory organ that accelerates diseases like diabetes, heart disease, cancer, and dementia.

- Rule of Thumb: Focus on abdominal fat, not just weight. "Don't chase weight. Chase waist."
- Longevity Marker: A waist-to-height ratio below 0.5 is strongly associated with a longer, healthier life.

These pillars ensure the body and brain have the time to repair and adapt to daily challenges.

5. Sleep Well: Repair, Recovery, and Renewal

Sleep is the body's master repair cycle. Adults need 7–8 hours of high-quality sleep. During deep sleep:

- The brain clears toxins (via the Glymphatic system).
- Memory and creativity improve.
- Hormones rebalance and immunity strengthens.

Expert Sleep Recommendations:

- Maintain consistent sleep timing.
- Ensure a dark, cool bedroom.
- Avoid screens 1–2 hours before bed.
- Get daylight exposure in the morning.

6. Resilience: Keep Stress Low and Manage Your Mind

Chronic stress accelerates aging at the cellular level by rapidly shortening telomeres (a marker of biological age). A calm mind supports a healthy body; emotional balance is as important as physical fitness.

Science-Backed Stress Reduction Tools:

- Meditation or mindfulness, gratitude practices.
- Yoga, pranayama, and deep breathing exercises.
- Daily walking and spending time in nature.
- Strong social connections

These habits ensure continuous learning, early detection, and strong social support.

7. Keep Your Brain Active and Engaged

Longevity is pointless without mental sharpness. New brain cells (neurogenesis) continue even in old age, provided we challenge the mind.

- Stimulation: Learn new skills, read, write, do music, puzzles, or memory games.
- Support: Maintain an anti-inflammatory diet, adequate sleep, and Omega-3 DHA/B12 levels.
- Socialize: Social interaction is key for cognitive health.

8. Prevent Disease Before It Starts

Early detection is the key to prevention. You can't manage what you don't measure.

- Tracking Metabolic Markers: Regular blood tests (HbA1c, fasting insulin, lipids).
- Structural Screening: DEXA scan for bone density; periodic heart screening (CT coronary calcium).
- Maintenance: Eye and dental care, and up-to-date vaccinations.

9. **Build Strong Social Connections and Purpose**

Studies from Harvard and Blue Zones show that warm, positive relationships are among the strongest predictors of long life—often more than diet or exercise. Connection reduces stress, supports mental health, and sharpens memory.

Live with Purpose: A strong sense of purpose, a passion, or a reason to wake up every morning fuels motivation and resilience. This mental framework adds years to life — and life to years.

10. **Use Supplements Wisely**

Even with a balanced diet, modern lifestyles can create nutrient gaps. Supplements can strengthen your foundation but are not a substitute for healthy eating.

- Consider: Vitamin D3, Magnesium, Omega-3 fatty acids, Vitamin K2, and a high-quality multivitamin—always under medical guidance.

11. **Prevent Accidents and Ensure Quick Recovery**

After age 70, falls and prolonged bed rest significantly threaten longevity.

- Safety: Improve balance and coordination (Tai Chi, yoga).
- Recovery: If illness occurs, prioritize quick recovery. Being bedridden for more than three days may cause significant muscle loss and complications.

By consistently embracing these habits—moving daily, eating smart, sleeping deeply, training your muscles and mind, managing stress, nurturing relationships, and performing preventive checks—you can dramatically increase both your lifespan and the quality of your final decades. This is the way to stay active, sharp, and vibrant until the very last day and enjoy every step of the life journey.

Learning:

The journey towards longevity is a marathon, not a sprint. It is a lifelong commitment to wellness. By following a comprehensive approach that includes healthy lifestyle, mindful nutrition, regular physical activity, monitoring health parameters, stress management, and strong social connections, we can significantly enhance our chances of living longer and remaining fit and vibrant throughout our lives.

Chapter 60

The fabulous Hormones of Happiness

Happiness hormones are special chemicals in our bodies—mainly neurotransmitters and hormones—that play a powerful role in creating feelings of joy, well-being, and emotional balance. Think of them as your body's natural "feel-good" messengers.

The four happiness hormones are:

1. Dopamine – The Reward Chemical

Released when you achieve something meaningful or experience pleasure. Dopamine fuels motivation, learning, and the satisfaction that comes from progress.

2. Serotonin – The Mood Stabilizer

This hormone helps regulate your mood, sleep, and appetite. Higher serotonin levels lead to feelings of calm and contentment while keeping stress at bay.

3. Oxytocin – The Love Hormone

This one blossoms through connection—during hugs, social bonding, or acts of affection. It promotes trust, empathy, and deep emotional bonds.

4. Endorphins – The Natural Painkillers

Released during exercise, laughter, or even after eating spicy food, Endorphins ease pain and create feeling of euphoria.

These four hormones send signals from the brain to the rest of the body, telling us how to feel. When they are flowing smoothly, we feel calm, confident, connected, and energized.

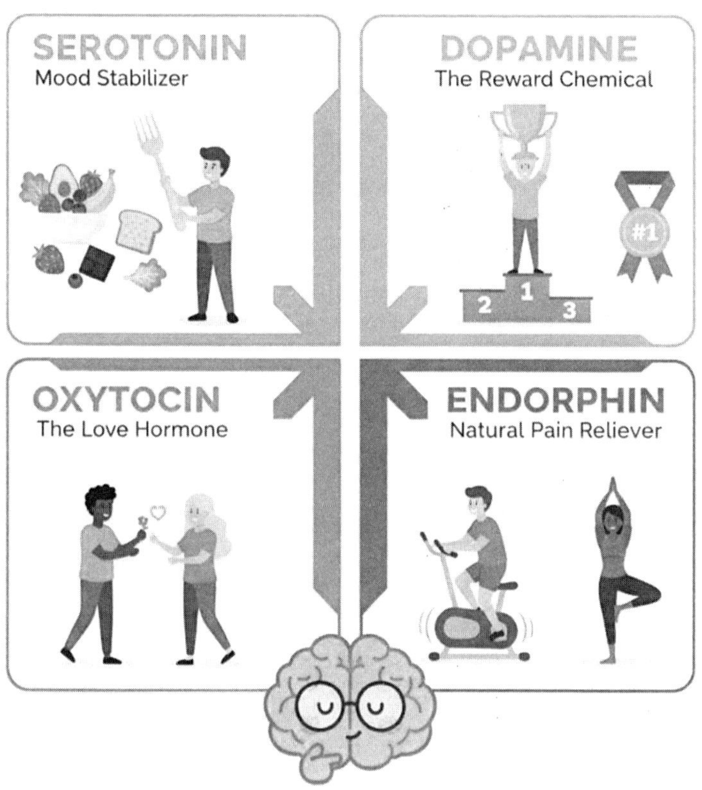

Where Are these Hormones produced?

While the brain is the main hub for these hormones, some are also produced in other organs.

- *Dopamine*: Produced in the brain, especially during goal achievement and pleasurable experiences.
- *Serotonin*: Produced mainly in the gut (about 90%) and the brain.

- *Oxytocin*: Produced in the hypothalamus and released by the pituitary gland.
- *Endorphins*: Produced in the brain and the nervous system in response to stress, pain, or joy.

How Can You Naturally Boost Happiness Hormones?

1. *Endorphins* work like natural painkillers.

To boost endorphins, Exercise regularly. Eat spicy foods.

2. *Serotonin* is your natural antidepressant. To increase serotonin, get sunlight, exercise outdoors. Eat tryptophan-rich foods. Practice positivity.

3. *Dopamine* gives you the rush of pleasure when you succeed or enjoy does something you enjoy. To boost dopamine, listen to music, set goals and achieve them, Exercise, Have your favourite sweets occasionally.

4. *Oxytocin* builds social bonds, trust, and emotional warmth.

To boost oxytocin, hug, kiss, or cuddle. Get a massage, Build close relationships.

Learning:

Happiness is not just a feeling—it is a science! Move more, laugh often, eat well, connect deeply and let your hormones work their magic.

Chapter 61

The Power of Belief - Placebo Effect

The placebo effect is a fascinating demonstration of the mind-body connection. Due to placebo effect, a person can experience real, measurable improvement in health condition after receiving a treatment that contained no active medicine. This benefit is triggered by the person's belief and expectation rather than by medicine.

Whether it's a sugar pill, saline injection, or even a fake surgery, the belief that one is receiving effective treatment can activate genuine physiological changes in the body. In short, healing begins not just with medicine, but often with the mind.

Does Science Support the Placebo Effect?

Decades of research in medicine, psychology, and neuroscience confirm that the placebo effect is real and measurable. Clinical trials consistently show that patients who believe they are receiving treatment often report significant improvements—even when that treatment is inert.

Brain imaging studies reveal that expectation and belief can trigger the release of powerful chemicals such as endorphins and dopamine, influencing mood, pain perception, and even immune function.

How Does the Placebo Effect Work?

1. Expectation and Belief

The mind anticipates healing, and the brain sets physiological processes in motion to match that belief.

2. Brain Chemistry Activation

Placebos can stimulate the brain to release feel-good chemicals like dopamine, serotonin, and endorphins, which reduce pain, lift mood, and enhance well-being.

3. Conditioned Responses

Over a period of time, the brain learns to associate pills, injections, or medical rituals with recovery—triggering healing responses, even when no active drug is present.

Who Uses the Placebo Principle in Practice?

While there are no "placebo specialists", certain healthcare professionals integrate placebo principles such as patient expectation, empathy, and therapeutic rituals into their care.

Pain Management Experts (Anaesthesiologists and Neurologists) understand that belief can powerfully influence pain perception, and they often use suggestion and environment to support recovery alongside conventional treatments.

Psychiatrists and Psychologists: Mental health conditions such as depression and anxiety are particularly responsive to the placebo effect. These professionals harness the mind-body link and therapeutic alliance to optimize healing.

Compassionate, Empathetic doctors who build strong relationships and trust with their patients often enhance the placebo response. Their genuine care can be just as healing as the medicine they prescribe.

Real-Life Examples: The Placebo Effect in Action

1. Pain Relief without Drugs

Example: In a study, patients who underwent fake knee surgeries (only skin incisions, no actual procedure) had pain relief equal to those who had real surgery—purely due to belief.

2. Boosting the Immune System

Example: People taking "flu-prevention" placebos often report fewer colds—belief appears to strengthen immune resilience.

3. Lowering Blood Pressure and Improving Heart Health

Example: Patients told they were taking heart meds experienced slowed heart rates and calmer moods.

4. Treating Depression and Anxiety

Example: Patients who believed they were on antidepressants reported significant improvement.

5. Improved Digestion and Gut Health

Example: IBS patients treated with placebos had symptom relief similar to those on real medicines.

6. Enhanced Athletic Performance

Example: Athletes who believed they had taken performance enhancers ran faster and lifted more, though they received only placebos.

7. Better Sleep without Pills

Example: Participants who thought they took sleeping pills reported deeper, more restful sleep—brain scans even showed slowed brain activity similar to actual sedatives.

8. Allergy Relief without Antihistamines

Example: Allergy sufferers taking placebo "antihistamines" still experienced symptom relief, purely from expectation.

Learning:

While the placebo effect does not cure major chronic diseases, it offers a powerful concept that the brain and body are deeply interconnected. Harnessing this connection—through trust, positive expectations, and supportive environments—can enhance healing, reduce symptoms, and improve quality of life.

Chapter 62

Yoga- The Body- Mind Connection

Yoga is the union of body, mind, and spirit. It integrates Yog asanas (postures), pranayama (breath control), and meditation. It nurtures inner peace, balance, and a deeper connection with oneself.

Benefits of Yoga

The benefits of yoga are profound—most of them internal and therapeutic. Regular practice helps relieve stress, anxiety, and mental tension. It is known to support the management of chronic conditions such as high blood pressure, diabetes, and arthritis. Yoga sharpens memory, enhances cognitive functions, and strengthens muscles, bones, and ligaments. It's not just a path to fitness—it's a journey toward holistic wellness.

Yoga vs. Traditional Exercise

While vigorous physical exercise can produce excessive free radicals in the body—potentially accelerating aging and tissue damage—yoga promotes slow, mindful movements that minimize such oxidative stress. Yoga works directly on specific organs and glands—for example, improving lung, heart, liver or spleen function and enhancing blood flow to the brain.

Patanjali's Ashtanga Yoga: The Eightfold Path

Around 300 B.C., the great sage Maharishi Patanjali offered the philosophy of yoga in the form of Ashtanga Yoga—a systematic path to self-realization. Today, this timeless wisdom is embraced worldwide as the science and art of life.

The eight limbs of Ashtanga Yoga are:

1. *Yamas (restraints):* Satya (truth), Ahimsa (non-violence), Asteya (non-stealing), Brahmacharya (celibacy/moderation), Aparigraha (non-possessiveness)
2. *Niyamas (observances):* Saucha (cleanliness), Santosha (contentment), Tapas (discipline), Swadhyaya (self-study), Ishwar Pranidhana (surrender to the divine)
3. *Asanas (physical postures)*
4. *Pranayama (control of breath)*
5. *Pratyahara (withdrawal of senses)*
6. *Dharana (concentration)*
7. *Dhyana (meditation)*
8. *Samadhi (state of blissful absorption or enlightenment)*

Over a period time, modern yoga masters have modified this ancient system, introducing new styles such as Bikram Yoga, Vinyasa Flow, Iyengar Yoga, and Power Yoga. In countries like the USA, yoga has grown into a massive wellness industry.

Important Yog asanas (Postures):

1-*Bhujangasana* (Cobra Pose)

Lie on your stomach with legs extended and palms placed under the shoulders. Inhale and slowly lift your head, chest, and upper abdomen while keeping the navel on the floor. Keep elbows close to the body, shoulders relaxed, and gaze forward or slightly upward. Hold for a few breaths, then exhale and return.

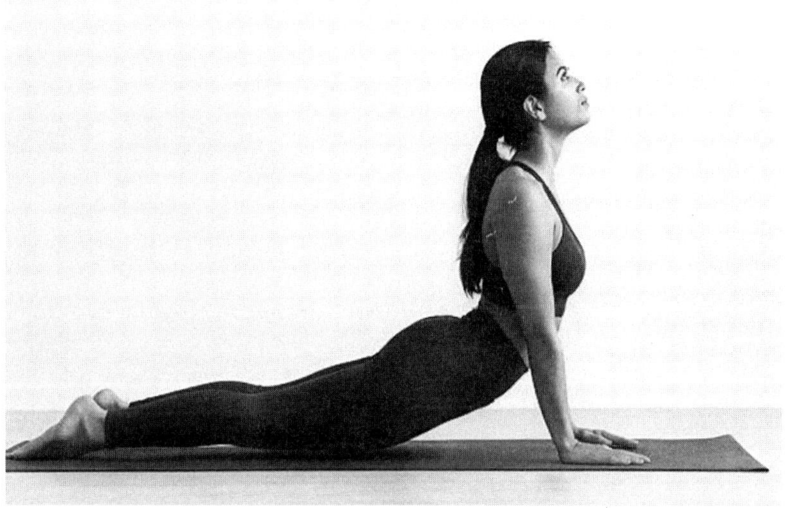

This asana strengthens the spine and opens the chest, improving spinal flexibility. As a result, respiratory and digestive processes are improved. It also increases lung capacity.

2-*Shalabhasana* (Locust Pose)

Lie flat on your stomach with arms alongside the body and palms facing down. Inhale and lift both legs together as high as possible without bending the knees, keeping arms and torso on the floor. Engage lower back and glute muscles, keeping the neck relaxed. Exhale and lower the legs gently.

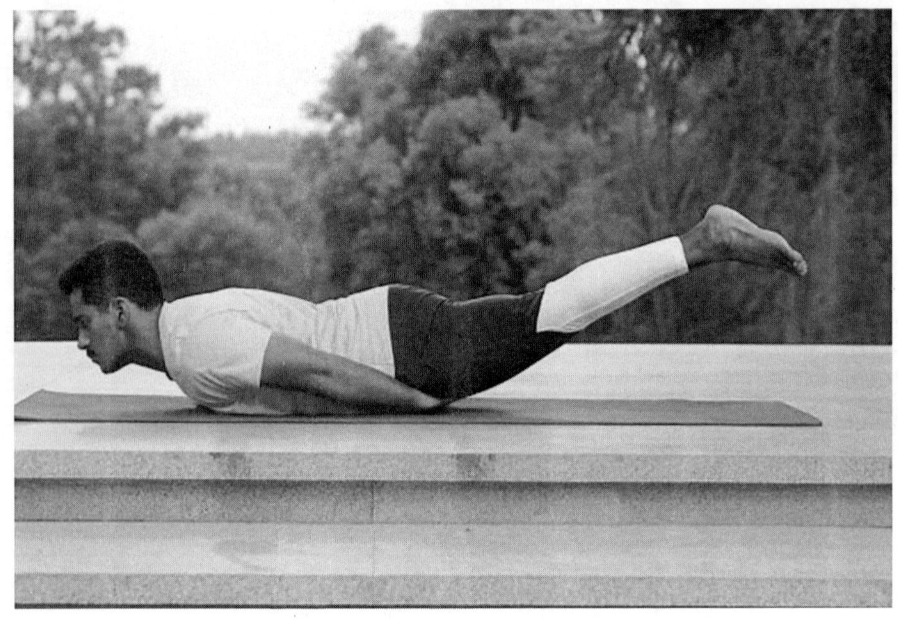

It strengthens lower back and stimulates abdominal organs.

3-*Pawanmuktasana* (Wind-Relieving Pose)

Lie on your back with legs extended. Bend both knees and draw them toward the chest, clasping them with your arms. Exhale and bring the head up, touching chin or nose to knees. Hold for a few breaths, then release gently.

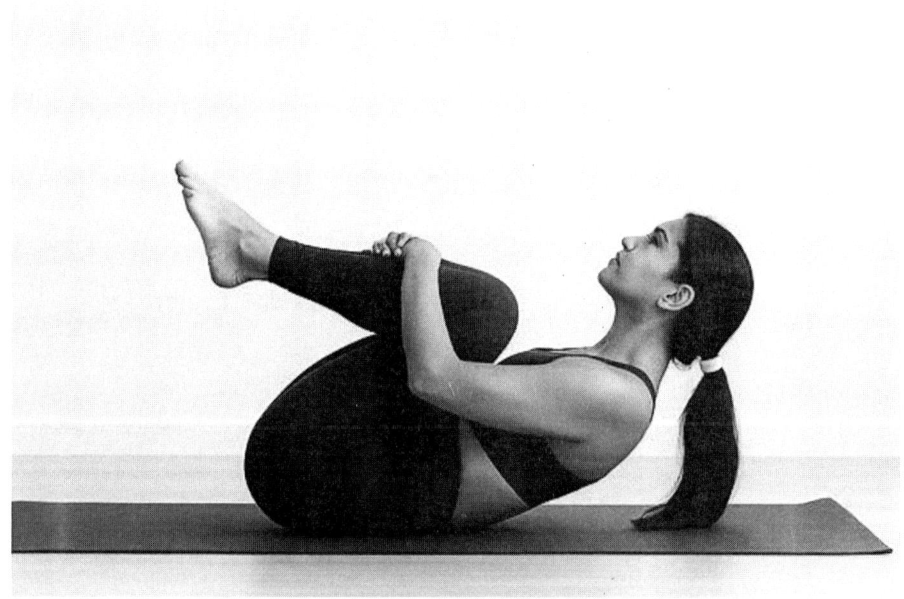

It relieves gas, aids digestion.

Strengthens lower back and hips.

4-*Trikonasana* (Triangle Pose)

Stand with feet wide apart and arms stretched sideways at shoulder level. Turn right foot out, left foot slightly in, and inhale. Exhale and bend sideways over the right leg, placing the right hand near the ankle or shin, and extend the left arm upward. Keep the torso open, then inhale and return.

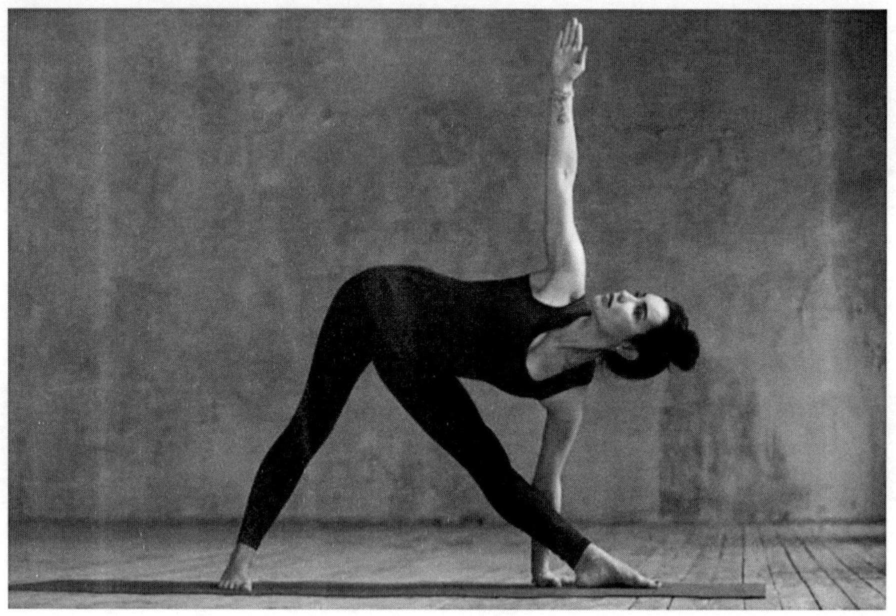

It improves spinal flexibility

Strengthens legs and core

5-*Padahastasana* (Hand-to-Foot Pose)

Stand straight with feet together. Inhale, raise both arms overhead, and while exhaling bend forward from the hips to touch your hands to the feet or floor. Keep knees straight and let the head move toward the knees. Stay for a few breaths, then inhale and return slowly.

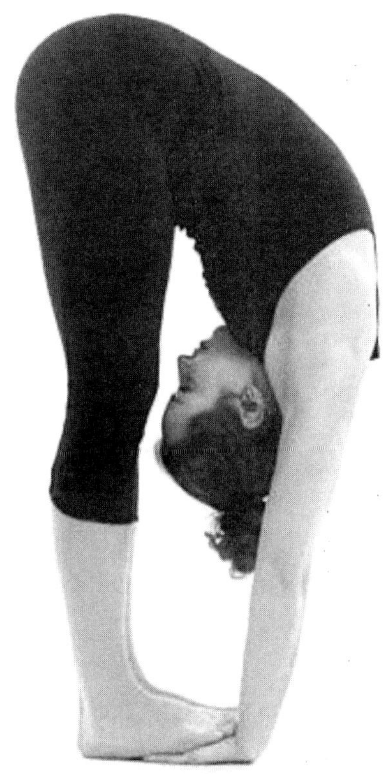

It Enhances blood flow to brain

Stretches hamstrings and spine

6-*Setu Bandhasana* (Bridge Pose)

Lie on your back with knees bent and feet hip-width apart, close to the hips. Place arms by your sides, palms down. Inhale and lift your hips upward, pressing into the feet and shoulders, keeping thighs parallel. Hold, then exhale and gently roll back down.

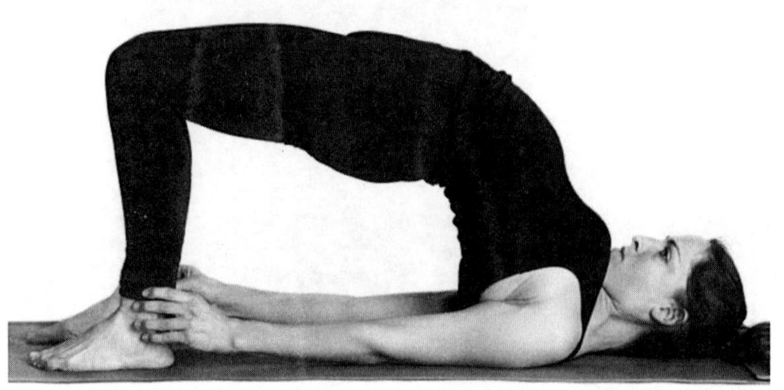

It strengthens back.

Opens chest and reduces thyroid imbalance

7-*Marjariasana* (Cat-Cow Stretch)

Come onto your hands and knees in a tabletop position. Inhale and arch your back downward, lifting the head and tailbone (cow stretch). Exhale and round your back upward, tucking the chin to the chest (cat stretch). Continue smoothly with the breath.

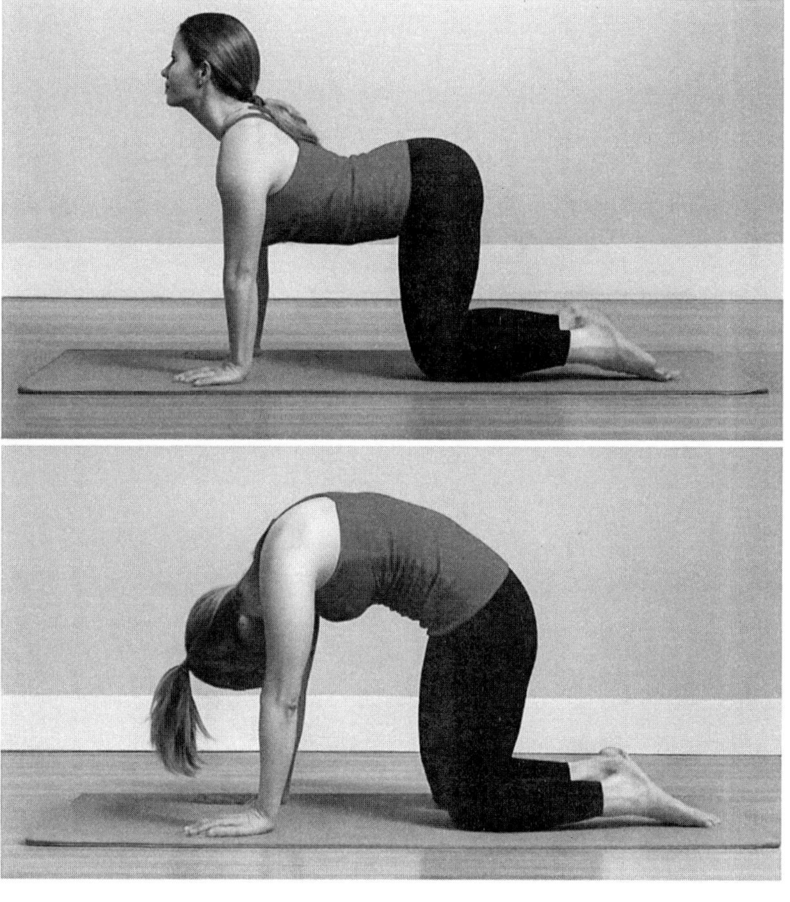

It Increases spinal flexibility. Improves blood circulation in spine.

8-*Adho Mukha Svanasana* (Downward-Facing Dog)

Start in a tabletop position, then tuck your toes and lift hips up and back. Straighten arms and legs to form an inverted "V" shape with the body. Keep the head between the arms and heels reaching toward the floor. Breathe steadily and hold.

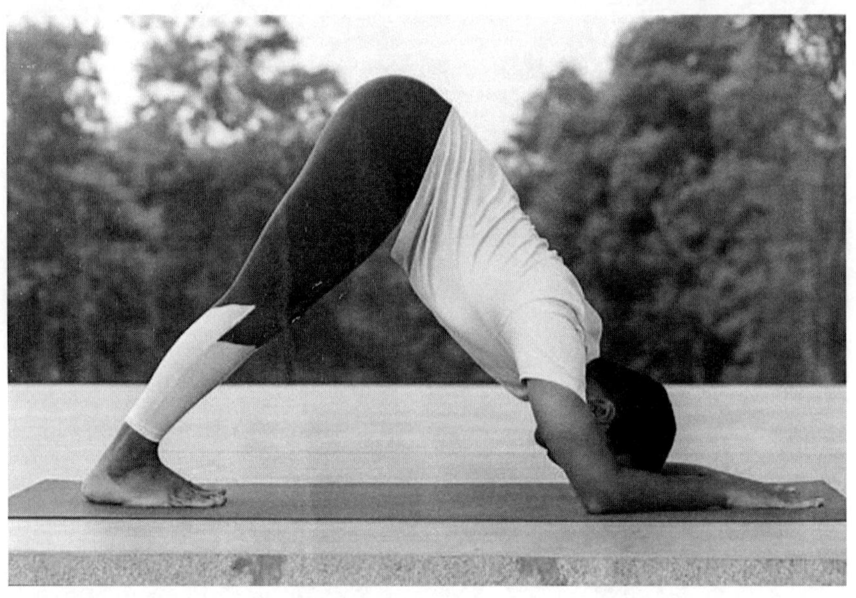

It Strengthens arms/shoulders

Relieves fatigue and energizes body

9-*Paschimottanasana* (Seated Forward Bend)

Sit with legs extended forward and spine straight. Inhale, raise both arms, then exhale and bend forward from the hips, reaching hands toward feet. Try to bring chest closer to thighs while keeping back lengthened. Hold for a few breaths, then release.

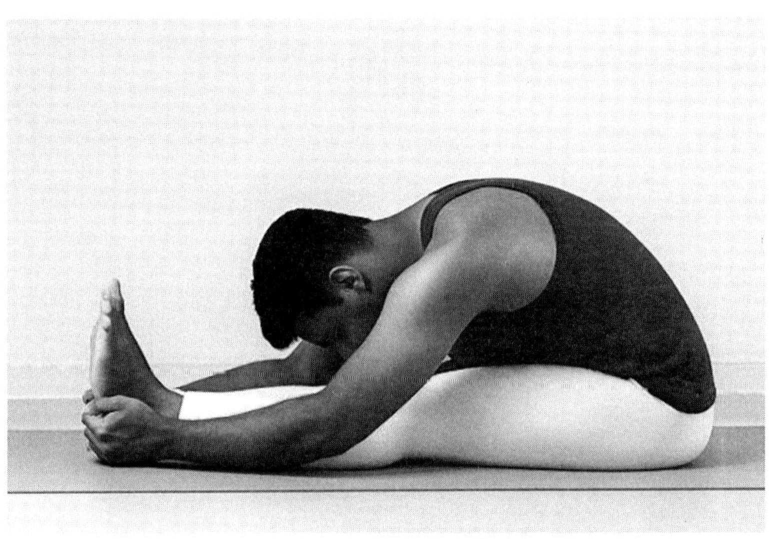

It Stretches spine, calms mind

Improves digestion and reduces belly fat

10-*Ardha Matsyendrasana* (Half Spinal Twist)

Sit with legs extended, then bend the right knee and place the foot outside the left thigh. Bend the left knee, bringing the heel near the right hip. Place right hand on the floor behind and left elbow outside the right knee. Inhale, lengthen spine; exhale, twist to the right.

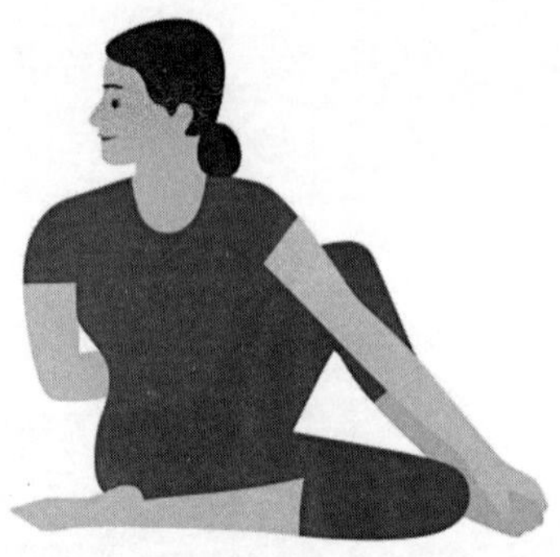

It Boosts spinal flexibility and detoxifies abdominal organs.

11-*Sarvangasana* (Shoulder Stand)

Lie flat on your back, arms by your side. Inhale and lift your legs up to 90°, then raise hips and back, supporting with palms on the lower back. Keep the body straight, chin slightly tucked, and gaze fixed on the chest. Hold steadily, then exhale and slowly roll down.

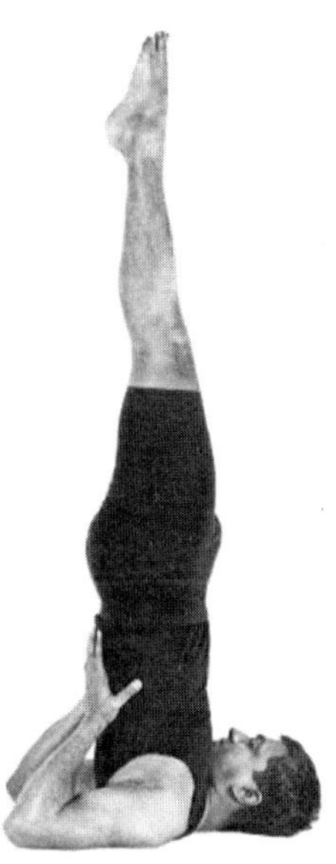

It is often called the queen of asanas because of its wide-ranging benefits. It improves blood circulation to the brain (since it is an inverted pose), stimulates thyroid and parathyroid glands, helping regulate metabolism and hormonal balance.

12-*Dhanurasana* (Bow Pose)

Lie on your stomach, bend your knees, and hold your ankles with your hands. Inhale and lift your chest and legs upward, pulling ankles gently to create a bow-like shape. Keep the head up and body balanced on the abdomen. Breathe steadily, then exhale and release.

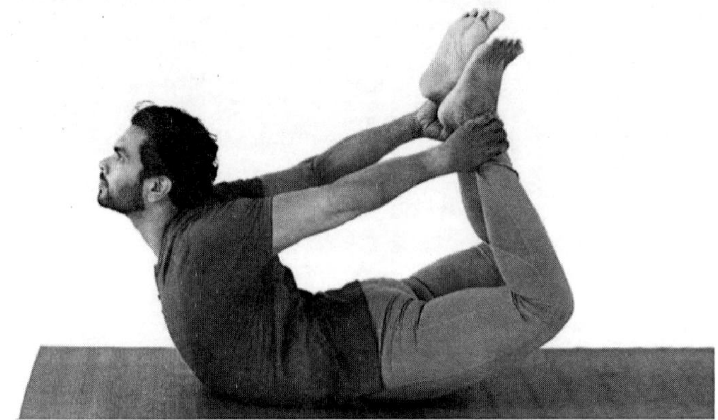

It strengthens back

Improves digestion and stimulates reproductive organs

Therapeutic Yoga:

Therapeutic Yoga is an evidence-based discipline that applies the principles and practices of yoga including postures (asanas) and breathing techniques (pranayama) to address specific physical, mental, and emotional health problems. It acts as a powerful complement to conventional medicine for managing conditions ranging from back pain and arthritis to hypertension and anxiety, ultimately improving overall quality of life.

1) Yoga for Hypertension

- Shavasana
- Makarasana
- Shashankasana
- Ardha Matsyendrasana
- Setu Bandhasana
- Viparita Karani

2) Yoga for Diabetes

- Vajrasana
- Mandukasana
- Ardhamatsyendrasana
- Dhanurasana
- Bhujangasana
- Paschimottanasana

3) Yoga for Back Pain

- Bhujangasana
- Ardha Shalabhasana
- Setu Bandhasana
- Marjarasana (Cat–Cow)
- Makarasana
- Shashankasana

4) Yoga for Knee Pain / Knee Joint Issues

- Tadasana
- Trikonasana
- Veerasana
- Ardha Kati Chakrasana
- Baddha Konasana

5) Yoga for Thyroid Function (Hypo/Hyper)

- Sarvangasana
- Halasana
- Matsyasana
- Bhujangasana
- Ustrasana
- Setu Bandhasana

6) Yoga for Anxiety / Depression

- Shavasana
- Balasana (Child's Pose)
- Viparita Karani
- Paschimottanasana
- Supta Baddha Konasana
- Marjarasana

The Philosophy behind Yoga

Yoga teaches us to cultivate the right mindset toward life. Excessive ambition is often the root of stress and unhappiness. Embracing simplicity and self-awareness leads to inner calm, healthier relationships, and reduced material cravings.

One of yoga's core principles is Karma Yoga—performing actions with detachment from their outcomes. This mindset fosters peace, clarity, and emotional balance. True yoga is about maintaining an inner stillness and blissful awareness even amidst dynamic action. With regular practice, one develops mindfulness, discipline, and deep self-transformation.

Yoga and Modern Science

Today, yoga is not just a spiritual pursuit—it is a scientifically validated health practice. Medical research increasingly supports yoga's effectiveness in treating and preventing various conditions, from anxiety to heart disease.

There is now a harmonious blend of Science, Yoga, and Spirituality. Western medicine is progressively embracing ancient yogic practices, acknowledging their transformative power. Yoga has become a bridge between physical health and inner peace—a complete system for total well-being.

Learning

Yoga is the best Preventive Medicine. It /is India's priceless gift to the world—a timeless tradition that offers physical vitality, mental clarity, emotional resilience, and spiritual awakening. Every individual should explore, learn, and experience the amazing benefits of this ancient toward health and longevity.

Chapter 63

The Science of Pranayama- A Magic Wand

The word Pranayama comes from the Sanskrit roots Prana (life force or breath) and Aayma (extension or control). Together, it means the conscious regulation of breath, a vital link between the body and mind. Through various techniques of inhalation, retention, and exhalation, pranayama helps harness and direct the flow of energy within the body.

Why Practice Pranayama?

Pranayama brings profound physical, mental, and spiritual benefits:

- Focuses awareness on breathing
- Reduces metabolic rate
- Enhances energy sensitivity
- Calms the mind and nervous system
- Expands awareness and consciousness
- Improves overall health and inner strength

Important Pranayama Techniques and Their Benefits

Anulom-Vilom (Alternate Nostril Breathing)

- Balances the logical (left brain) and emotional (right brain) hemispheres.
- Harmonizes the sympathetic (fight-or-flight) and parasympathetic (rest-and-digest) nervous systems.
- Reduces stress, lowers metabolic rate, and promotes tranquillity.

- Therapeutic for asthma, bronchitis, nasal allergies, high blood pressure, and diabetes.
- Clears pranic blockages and balances Ida and Pingala nadis, enabling flow in Sushumna Nadi—key for meditation and spiritual awakening.

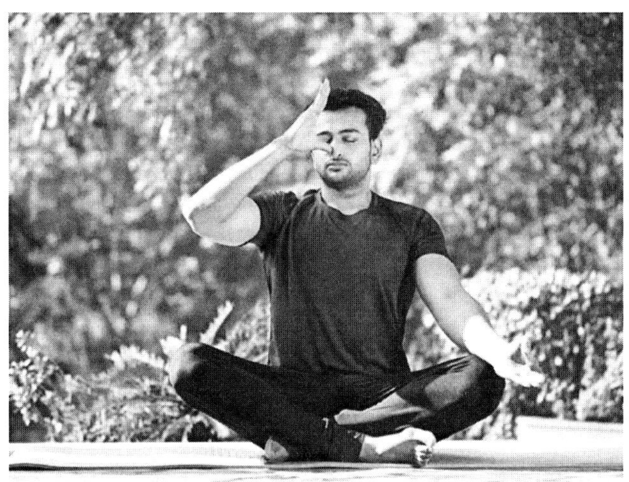

Chandra Anulom-Vilom aids in weight gain, while Surya Anulom-Vilom supports weight loss.

Kapalbhati (Skull-Shining Breath)

- Rapid, forceful exhalations and passive inhalations (up to 100–120 per minute).

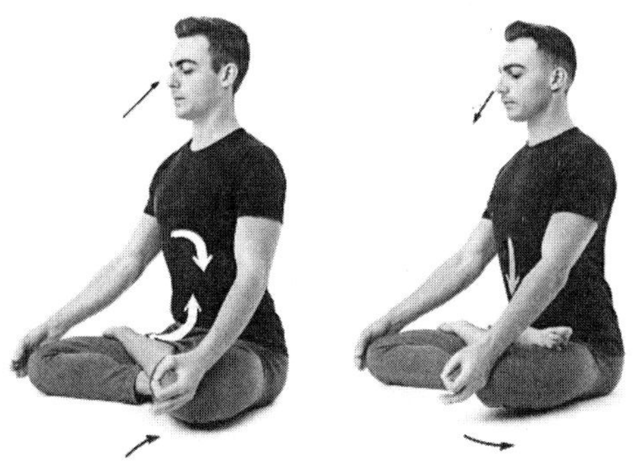

- Massages abdominal organs, improves digestion, and enhances oxygen supply.
- Stimulates endocrine and exocrine glands and sharpens memory.
- Beneficial for obesity, diabetes, thyroid issues, and respiratory problems.
- Caution: Avoid if you have high BP, heart disease, slip disc, or are pregnant/menstruating.

Ujjayi (Ocean Breath)
- Slows breath rate from 15 to 4 per minute, enhancing vagal tone and parasympathetic activity.
- Reduces hypertension, anxiety, and stress.
- Strengthens the epiglottis, improves vocal quality, and relieves throat conditions.
- Brings spiritual focus to the throat centre and promotes inner calm.
- Great for thyroid issues, asthma, chronic colds, and snoring.

Bhramari (Humming Bee Breath)
- Restores nervous and endocrine balance.
- Enhances vocal resonance and induces a meditative state.
- Quickly alleviates anger, anxiety, tension, and frustration.
- Soothes throat ailments and nurtures spiritual awareness.

Bhastrika (Bellows Breath)
- Energizes the body and burns fat by increasing metabolic rate.
- Builds respiratory capacity and purifies the blood.
- Balances the three doshas—Vata, Pitta, and Kapha.

- Helps release negative emotions and stress by regulating the nervous and endocrine systems.

Sitali & Sitkari (Cooling Breaths)

- Reduce body temperature and basal metabolic rate.
- Relax muscles and calm the nervous system.
- Help with allergies, anxiety, and heat-related conditions.
- Expand sensory perception and lung capacity.

How Pranayama Influences Involuntary Body Functions

Many essential body processes like heartbeat, digestion and hormone secretion—are regulated by the Autonomic Nervous System (ANS) and occur automatically without our conscious efforts. However, breathing process is unique: it is both involuntary and voluntary. This dual nature makes breathing a powerful tool to influence otherwise automatic functions.

How Pranayama Helps Control the Autonomic Nervous System

- Activates the parasympathetic nervous system (relaxation mode)
- Reduces stress hormones like cortisol and adrenaline
- Improves heart rate variability – a sign of nervous system resilience
- Stimulates the Vagus nerve, which controls many internal organs
- Influences hormone secretion, digestion, and immune response

Ujjayi Pranayama: Gateway to Autonomic Control

- Activates the parasympathetic system, reducing stress and anxiety

- Enhances vagal tone for better mood, digestion, and cardiovascular function
- Promotes coherent heart rhythms and emotional balance
- Brings conscious control over breath—an involuntary function

How to Practice Ujjayi Pranayama

1. Sit comfortably, keeping your spine straight and shoulders relaxed.
2. Breathe deeply a few times to centre yourself.
3. Constrict the throat slightly (as if whispering or fogging a mirror with your mouth closed).
4. Inhale slowly through the nose with the throat constricted—producing a soft ocean-like sound.
5. Exhale slowly through the nose with the same throat control and sound.
6. Focus on the sound and breath, using it as your meditative anchor.
7. Continue for 5–10 minutes, gradually increasing with comfort.
8. End by returning to normal breathing and sitting quietly for a moment.

Therapeutic Pranayama

Therapeutic Pranayama focusses on regulating the *prana* (life force) through conscious control of the breath. It shifts Nervous system from a "fight-or-flight" (sympathetic) response to a relaxing and restorative (parasympathetic) state, thereby reducing stress, anxiety, lowering blood pressure, improving respiratory capacity, and calming the mind.

1) For Hypertension

- Anuloma Viloma (Alternate Nostril Breathing)
- Bhramari Pranayama (Bee Breath / Humming Breath)

- Sheetali Pranayama (Cooling Breath)
- Suryabhedana Pranayama (Right-nostril Breathing)

2) For Asthma / Lung-related Issues

- Anuloma Viloma (Alternate Nostril Breathing)
- Bhastrika Pranayama (Bellows Breath)
- Kapalabhati Pranayama (Skull-Shining Breath / Cleansing Breath)
- Ujjayi Pranayama (Ocean Breath)

3) For Thyroid

- Ujjayi Pranayama
- Bhramari Pranayama
- Nadi Shodhana Pranayama (Alternate Nostril Breathing)
- Suryabhedana Pranayama

4) For Anxiety / Depression

Bhramari Pranayama.

- Anuloma Viloma (Alternate Nostril Breathing
- Yogic (Diaphragmatic) Deep Breathing / slow deep breathing
- Ujjayi Pranayama

Learning:

Pranayama is a powerful key to unlock vitality, mental clarity, emotional balance, and spiritual awareness. It empowers you to influence involuntary body systems through the conscious act of breathing. With regular practice, you will experience, inner peace and bliss, greater emotional stability, spiritual progress and expansion of awareness. In essence, Pranayama is not just breath control—it is life mastery.

Chapter 64

Bliss of Gratitude & Forgiveness

Gratitude is the appreciation that arises when we acknowledge the gifts—both big and small—that life bestows upon us. When we consciously turn our attention toward what we have, rather than what we lack, a quiet joy begins to blossom within us, fostering a deep sense of contentment and resilience.

Forgiveness, on the other hand, gently removes the hurts and resentments that may have taken root in our hearts. It is a conscious act of releasing emotional burdens—a liberating choice we make for ourselves. Holding onto anger and bitterness only scorches the one who holds it. Forgiveness is a courageous act of letting go, allowing us to heal and move forward with a lighter heart.

Everyday Blessings We Often Overlook

Here are a few blessings from God that we often take for granted:

-The simple gift of being alive and having a healthy body

-A safe shelter, nourishing food, and a clean environment

-The ability to see vibrant sunsets, hear a loved one's voice, taste a delicious meal, feel the warmth of the sun, and smell fresh rain

-Relationships with family and friends that offer love, support, and companionship

Cultivating Gratitude: Simple Daily Practices

Gratitude is a powerful practice that can profoundly enhance your well-being. Here are some easy ways to incorporate it into your daily life:

-*Morning Reflection*: Before getting out of bed, think of one thing you're grateful for—be it the warmth of your blanket, a good night's sleep, or the promise of a new day.

-*Evening Review*: Before sleeping, recall three specific blessings from your day—a compliment, a beautiful sunset, or a task you completed.

-*Say "Thank You" Sincerely*: When someone helps you, pause, make eye contact, and express genuine appreciation.

-*Kindness Without Expectation*: Show gratitude by doing something kind for others—hold a door, let someone go ahead in line, or offer a heartfelt compliment.

-*Incorporate Gratitude into Prayer or Meditation*:

These small, intentional acts can shift your mindset from scarcity to abundance, helping you appreciate the richness of life.

How Gratitude Alleviates Stress

Stress often stems from focusing on problems, losses, or disappointments. Gratitude shifts your attention from a "deficit mindset" to an "abundance mindset." By deliberately noticing and appreciating the good, you train your brain to focus on the positive—breaking the cycle of negativity.

Gratitude lowers cortisol levels, promoting relaxation and calming the nervous system.

It's linked to reduced symptoms of depression and anxiety
Physical benefits include better sleep, improved immunity, and reduced risk of heart disease

A Prayer of Gratitude

Supreme Power of the Universe,

With a heart full of gratitude, I thank you for the gift of life, for the joy that fills my days, and for the comforts that surround me. Thank You for the love and warmth of a caring family—for their presence, support, and kindness that make every moment special. I am grateful for simple joys—laughter shared peace in quiet moments, and the strength to face each new day. Thank You for the opportunities to grow, to love, and to give back to the world. May I always cherish what I have, appreciate those around me, and find happiness in the present moment. Guide me to be a source of kindness, understanding, and positivity, so I may share the blessings I've received with others. With a heart full of thanks, I embrace this day.

Forgiveness: A Path to Inner Peace

Forgiving those who have hurt us—and seeking forgiveness from those whom we have hurt—are powerful ways to reduce emotional and mental stress. Forgiveness releases us from the grip of negative emotions. Holding onto anger, resentment, or revenge keeps us in a constant state of "fight or flight," harming both mind and body
Guilt, shame, and regret from hurting others can weigh heavily; seeking forgiveness helps release these burdens, restore relationships, and improve self-esteem.

Forgiveness—both giving and receiving—is about letting go of the past to move forward with peace. It's an act of self-care that frees us from emotional chains.

Bedtime Prayer to Forgive Others

Supreme Power of the Universe,

Tonight, I release the weight of pain and bitterness from my heart. Those who have hurt me—knowingly or unknowingly—I choose to forgive. I may not forget the past, but I refuse to let it hold power over my peace and happiness. Grant me the strength to let go of resentment, to heal from past wounds, and to move forward with love and wisdom. May my heart be free from anger, and may I find peace in understanding that we are all imperfect, learning, and growing. With a heart open to forgiveness and peace, I rest tonight.

Bedtime Prayer for Seeking Forgiveness

Supreme Power of the Universe,

Tonight, I reflect on my words and actions. If I have hurt anyone—knowingly or unknowingly, in thought, word, or deed—I ask for their forgiveness. May their hearts find peace, and may any pain I've caused be healed with time, understanding, and love. Grant me the wisdom to recognize my mistakes, the strength to make amends, and the humility to grow into a kinder, more compassionate person. Help me forgive others too, releasing any burdens of anger or regret. With a heart open to forgiveness and peace, I rest tonight.

Seeking Forgiveness from Oneself

Supreme Power of the Universe,

Please forgive me for the hurt and pain I've caused to myself—physically, emotionally, and mentally. I willingly let go of the past. I will not repeat the same mistakes. I will care for myself with love and compassion. Thank You for Your mercy and grace. I receive Your forgiveness in full faith.

Learning

When we are grateful for the present moment and the good that surrounds us, it becomes easier to release the grip of past grievances. Similarly, when we forgive, we create space within our hearts for joy and appreciation to flourish. Together, gratitude and forgiveness create a sanctuary within us—a place of peace, healing, and acceptance.

Universal Prayer for Health & Happiness

ॐ सर्वे भवन्तु सुखिनः
सर्वे सन्तु निरामयाः ।
सर्वे भद्राणि पश्यन्तु
मा कश्चिद् दुःखभाग् भवेत ॥
ॐ शान्तिः शान्तिः शान्तिः ॥

"May all beings be happy.
May all be free from illness.
May everyone see and experience what is good and auspicious.
May no one suffer or be touched by sorrow.
May there be peace, peace, peace."